# The 7 Secrets of
## Healthy
# HAPPY PEOPLE

# The **7** Secrets of Healthy HAPPY PEOPLE

## Improve Your Mood, Emotions, Energy, Weight, and Life!

# ERLEEN TILTON

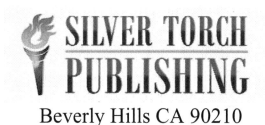

Beverly Hills CA 90210

The 7 Secrets of Healthy, Happy People: Improve Your Mood, Emotions, Energy, Weight, and Life!

Copyright © 2015 by Erleen Tilton

www.the7secretsbook.com
info@the7secretsbook.com

Published by Silver Torch Publishing
www.SilverTorchPublishing.com

Library of Congress Control Number 2015906744
ISBN 978-1-942707-06-6

Cover design by David T. Fagan and Carli Smith.

Printed in the United State of America.

# TABLE OF CONTENTS

# ACKNOWLEDGEMENTS

Many thanks to several people in order to bring this book to you.

Thank you, David Fagan, for inspiring me to share these things that I have learned and applied over the last 30 plus years.

Thank you, Jill Fagan, for taking on the task of bringing this book to life!

Thank you, my dear friends who have shared your stories within this book and for those who have shared your stories not included here. Your experiences are empowering and so helpful for others in their journey to wellness.

Thank you, my wonderful husband, Bill, you have been my continual support in my journey to wellness as well as my journey in helping others find wellness too.

Thank you, my wonderful family for your love and support – you are all my dearest treasures! This is written for you most of all!

But most of all, I thank my Father in Heaven for teaching me as a young mother how wellness can be found within his creations. I have felt from the start that my real source of education came from on high. I will ever be grateful for the bounties of blessings I have received as I have come to understand the power of wellness through God's creations!

# PREFACE

As a young mother, just after having my second child, life was wonderful…or was it? With a two-year old daughter and a son a few months old, my challenges seemed overwhelming! I had no energy, dealt with severe pollen allergies and migraine headaches, and my neck and back aches were constant and required frequent visits to a chiropractor. I then began feeling pain in my knees. Was it arthritis at age 21? Then the development of breast lumps…five…eight…a dozen. I stopped counting because it was depressing! I was suffering with so many ailments that I had only thought possible for the elderly. Why me? What was wrong?

I began reaching out…scared of what might happen if I went to the doctor. I was not getting a mastectomy at my age. I was not going to consider this. I had heard from our chiropractor's wife of a black salve so I decided to give it a try on one of the lumps. Well, it removed it BIG time. It left a huge hole at the side of one breast close to my under arm. I realized that if I kept this up, I'd be giving myself a double mastectomy all on my own. What next? I decided to go and get a mammogram just to be safe. The MD did notice the huge scar, but then he told me the lumps were benign and that I had to omit four things for life: coffee, tea, cola drinks, and chocolate. You got it – caffeine! This medical doctor shared with me that women are more sensitive to caffeine and are much more at risk for breast cancer. Well, I decided from that day forward these would be forever avoided. I can say I have held to that almost perfectly.

During this period of time I was also introduced to a NMD (Naturopathic Medical Doctor) initially for back and neck adjustments. During these visits, he would notice certain things. One time, he asked if I had a headache, and I admitted I did. How did he know? He said that my temperature was elevated! Did you know your temperature rises when you have a headache? I didn't. He offered to administer some tests to find out the cause to some of the issues I was trying to work through. Of course I consented. What did I have to lose? I was a young mother, and I didn't know what life would look like in a year or two if I didn't start feeling better – it truly scared me. I didn't like feeling so physically and emotionally run down.

Tests were run – hair and blood samples – and the lab work revealed disorders, some of which I was completely unfamiliar with: hypoglycemia, anemia, valley fever, colitis, extreme vitamin deficiency, and my body was high in toxic drugs, barbiturates in fact. Where did this come from?

What now? I needed a new plan for life. I wasn't really ready for it, but I did have several things going for me. I had a huge desire to get well, I had a mentor I communicated with often to guide me through, and I was given an outlined program of how I could succeed! So first, here was the regimen…a four-part system for healing, one that literally saved my life!

Step one was a whole foods diet. I was severely lacking nutrition, so the first part of this was to remove all the processed foods, refinement, milk products, breads – yes all breads even whole-grain breads – from my diet. What was left? He smiled…loads of raw, fresh fruits and vegetables, some lightly steamed, whole grains (cooked or sprouted), whole cooked beans, raw seeds and nuts, fertile eggs, lean white meats on occasion…foods full of nutrition, fiber, enzymes and more! So the following day I arose for breakfast. No bread or cereal, but that was okay, I'd cook some cracked wheat. Yes, but no milk, no sugar! That morning was tough. I think my tears helped some of the food slide down that day. BUT I was determined to get well!

After a few days though, it was just too much. I was starving, and I felt deprived all the time. I called up this naturopath and asked the question, "How long do I have to stick with this diet?" I will never forget the long pause on the other end and then the quiet but firm answer that was life changing, "Forever if you want to be healthy." That's not what I wanted to hear! But what he helped me understand was that if I were to go back to my old way of eating I would never get well, or stay well – and I really did want to get well.

I changed my tone and decided to focus on foods I could have – not foods I couldn't have – and this made all the difference in the world! There are loads of healthy foods available. It wasn't a matter of going without, just a matter of focusing on foods that would benefit me and make me whole again.

About two months into it, I stopped by the grocery store close to lunch time – big mistake – big lesson! I was hungry, and home was twenty minutes away after shopping was over. Passing by the bakery, I saw a huge cinnamon swirl. I had never eaten one before, and I decided that I had been doing so well and was feeling so much better that just this once wouldn't hurt. I plowed in and ate the whole thing! I didn't even finish up my shopping before I felt that old me coming back again…no energy, headache coming on, depression, extreme fatigue, emotionally strung out. By the time I got to my car, I was crying, I was so upset…how could this make such a HUGE difference in the way I felt? But it did, and I didn't like it! I decided that I would NEVER go back to that world. It would never be worth feeling that bad again! I could feel the night-and-day difference in nourishing foods and processed foods within just a few minutes!

Step two was cleansing. He put me on several cleanses. One was a very expensive 30-day detox with pills taken in a strict format for purging the toxic drugs from my system. The worst (but probably the best) was a three-day lemon and water cleanse. I thought I would die from that one…literally! Talk about no energy – it pulled every ounce of strength I had to consume only water and fresh lemon juice – nothing else for three whole days! I also did some fresh juice fasting for days here and there at other times. And on top of that, I did colonics too – twice-weekly then weekly for several weeks. Wow…he showed me the calcium deposits that came out of my colon. Some of them were the size of green peas and when they dried out, they became "chalk" like what I used in school to write on the chalkboard! Cleansing the toxins out of my system was a necessary step of healing! My body was not functioning because I was so full of toxicity!

Step three, was building. He gave me more supplements than I thought was possible to take in one handful…vitamins, minerals, digestive aids, herbs – it seemed like something for everything. And they were expensive too, adding up to between $250 and $300 monthly. For those of you who have lost track of time, back thirty years ago, this was MORE than my mortgage payment. Was this worth it? Could I afford it? But how could I NOT afford it? We would just have to come up with it somehow – and we did. I soon realized that yes, diet is the foundation and must be full of nutrition to supply the body with the needed nutrients in order to function properly. The toxicity must be removed as well, but to accelerate the process, concentrated nutrition in the form of whole food supplements were absolutely necessary. In other words, these were necessary to pull me out of the bottom of a pit...and they did!

Step four was repair or support. This NMD helped me understand the power of nature's medicines vs. the dangers of synthetic medicines with the chemical reactions and side effects. Even if I were to do the first three steps perfectly, using synthetic medicines would not provide the optimal results I needed. So I began a new adventure in plant medicines, which had just recently been introduced through another chiropractor's wife with the black salve and other home remedies she was suggesting. I could see the value of herbal medicines for specific areas that needed repair or support, and I found great results with the myriad of recommendations made. This also spurred me into a new area of learning all I could.

Within a five- to six-month period, I was an entirely different person! No more migraines or even headaches (and I can honestly say I haven't had more than two headaches within these past thirty-plus years), all the breast lumps disappeared, no more depression or mood swings, I had loads of energy, my bowels were moving, and my health was a complete turnaround! About two years later, I realized I'd had no more pollen allergies since the time of changes. I had always thought it was the grass and the blossoms creating my allergies, but it was just my polluted system being stirred up in rebellion that was creating those symptoms.

I learned that almost all dysfunction, disorder, and disease can actually be traced to two main things: lack of nutrition for the body to function optimally and too much toxicity, which inhibits proper function and order. That's it! In almost any given situation, although I do realize that there are other factors influencing our health, these areas are foundational. Given the proper nutrition with whole foods and balanced supplements, and cleansing out the toxicity, your body and my body have the ability to function normally and optimally.

I learned that whole foods and medicines found in nature were true and powerful gifts of love from God to give us LIFE and ENERGY – instead of sickness and misery – but they will only help us if we partake of them!

The depression, crying spells, colon problems, valley fever, breast lumps, allergies, arthritis...both emotional and physical issues...were simply due to the fact that I had been largely ignoring the gifts in nature and had been embracing man's inferior creations that were lacking the tools my body desperately needed...and I was suffering because of this.

It's not a wonder that there are many, many people in our world today suffering as I was...and worse! After finding my new found health, I would often look around and think, "Why doesn't everyone know this? Why is this such a secret in our society? Why have I not been taught this before? Why aren't we all taught this?"

I learned the power of change. Even though it was extremely hard to go "cold turkey", just turn and move in an entirely different direction, I know I would have never seen the results had I tried to do it gradually. I needed to do it ALL at once...whole foods, cleansing, building, and target support from nature in order to get well. I had to know where the fence was. Without that, I would have never been able to make these changes! And even more important, I knew that if I wanted to permanently change my outcome or results, I had to PERMANENTLY CHANGE MY HABITS. There was NO other way! My habits were ruling and ruining me. I had to make some changes...permanently!

This started my journey of education in wellness, prevention, optimal health, and freedom from sickness and disease. I began learning all I could as I continued to raise my beautiful children...six in all eventually. I took classes, I researched (even in a day without internet), I began creating a cookbook full of recipes for healthy, wholesome foods – because nothing like that was out there at that time – and I published my first in 1983, *Naturally, It's Better!* I began teaching classes on better eating, organic gardening, herbal first-aid, then writing books in those areas as well. Speaking at many venues was such a joy! I was so shy as a youth, but I now had passion and a purpose – I had renewed health, and I loved sharing my newfound knowledge of wellness with the world.

I learned, however, that as amazing as this four-part formula is, it was not complete. We must embrace three more important areas that influence total wellness, and once you understand all of these and the secrets that lie within each one, you will understand that these are key for creating a healthier, happier life physically, emotionally, mentally, and spiritually.

In the early 2000s, I became more intent on teaching these well-kept secrets that I had been learning. I created my own three-day mountain retreats and full-day herbal workshops. I also became introduced to essential oils and found some great successes with their use. But it wasn't until the latter part of 2010 that I truly understood the power of essential oils that can come with superior therapeutic quality and purity. These particular essential oils provided far more results than I had ever seen in my past thirty years of study and experience with herbals, homeopathics, or any other oils, and I was amazed. There were more well-kept secrets that were being unfolded before me. Why was I just learning about them now?

I am sharing with you an accumulation of over thirty years of important information that will surely enlighten you. But there's more! Hopefully this will certainly not be the end of your quest for wellness, but will either be a good start or it will better solidify your understanding of nature and God's plan for his children…enjoying health for life!

**DISCLAIMER:** Throughout this book, there are statements made which have not been evaluated by the Food and Drug Administration. These are not meant to diagnose, treat, cure, or take the place of professional advice from a physician. You are always encouraged to seek professional advice for your family as needed.

# INTRODUCTION

Before addressing these chapters containing The 7 Secrets, let's look at some pieces of information that will set the foundation. These areas will possibly help you see things in a whole different light than you've ever seen before. Focus on the message of each of these areas.

## EASTERN MEDICINE VS. WESTERN MEDICINE

Eastern Medicine differs from Western Medicine in many ways as you will see below. Because many of us have been raised with the Western Medicine mentality, most often when we go to address wellness modalities and nature's medicines, we still have the tendency to think like the Western Medicine mentality and act on crisis and symptoms.

You need to understand the difference between these two methods and realize that if acting upon symptoms and treatments doesn't give long-term benefits, you shouldn't mimic this approach! Think as Eastern Medicine does in order to find true success in wellness by keeping your focus on the root cause and prevention of disease, dysfunction, and disorder instead of on crisis and symptom treatments. Then, and only then, can you experience true long-term wellness.

Here is an illustration that will help you further understand this:

## EASTERN MEDICINE

**FOCUS:** Root cause and prevention

**HEALTH:** A state of well being in which the body is vital, balanced & adaptive to its environment.

## WESTERN MEDICINE

**FOCUS:** Crisis and symptom management

**HEALTH:** Absence of disease, pain, defect, or symptoms of illness (no theory of health).

| EASTERN MEDICINE | WESTERN MEDICINE |
|---|---|
| **THE PHYSICIAN:** As a gardener or assistant: to cultivate life, to help patient get/stay well. | **THE PHYSICIAN:** As mechanic: to fix what is broken. |
| **PREVENTION:** The major thrust of medicine, Chinese doctors are only paid if people stay well. | **PREVENTION:** Not the primary concern, actively discouraged by original insurance plans. |
| **TREATMENT:** Preventing illness by balancing disharmonious energy and counseling lifestyle management. | **TREATMENT:** Curing named disease and suppressing symptoms through drugs or surgery. |
| **SCIENCE OF MEDICINE FOCUS:**<br>• giving plant ingredients to the body, still coupled with their natural, organic carriers<br>• the body can do the extracting and regulating<br>• studies show that the human body recognizes them as whole foods and thereby extracts only what it needs | **SCIENCE OF MEDICINE FOCUS:**<br>• extracting and controlling the active ingredients in plants<br>• converting them to drug substances to halt disease<br>• extraction is done in a laboratory, bypassing the body's participation<br>• body often reacts to these synthetics and isolated chemicals by manifesting side-effect |

If the Western medical approach is on symptom management, are we mimicking it with nature's medicines as we encounter situations? For example, if you have a headache, what do you reach for? The Western mentality reaches for some form of pain reliever.

If you've been schooled in nature's medicines, you might reach for peppermint or frankincense essential oil or a blend that is effective for pain, and apply it. That oftentimes gives relief within a few minutes and is awesome!

However, have you questioned the cause of the headache and how to prevent getting a headache to begin with? Most people simply think headaches are part of life. They think headaches come without feeling any responsibility for having "created" it. They don't know they can possibly avoid one in the future.

The truth is there are several possible causes of headaches, minor or major:

- Processed foods: refined sugar, refined flour, and refined oils can become glue in your gut because they have no fiber or nutrients, so they can sit there and decay
- Chemical triggers such as artificial colors, flavors, sweeteners, preservatives, and other additives are often huge culprits
- Bulk foods: too much meat, potatoes, and breads in the gut all at once (lacking adequate enzymes)
- Soft drinks, sport drinks, energy drinks – these are big
- Structural issues: spinal alignment is out of balance, and you are in need of a chiropractor
- Compacted colon: even if you are having regular bowel movements, you may have pockets in your colon that are decaying with toxicity being continually reabsorbed back into your bloodstream
- Lack of water: not just lack of fluids here, but lack of pure water to allow your system the natural cleansing that is required

If you get to the root of the cause, then you can have a starting point to prevent future challenges. If you don't look to the cause and just "treat the symptom," then you fall into the trap of the Western Medicine mentality. And if that system is broken, then we need to relearn how to take a whole different approach and follow the Eastern Medicine path.

## PURE THERAPEUTIC GRADE ESSENTIAL OILS

For thousands of years, oils extracted from aromatic plants have been recognized as one of the most superior and effective medicines known to mankind.[1] Many of the books in the Holy Bible mention essential oils or the plants that produce them. These were considered holy ointments and medicines in their purest form given by God to demonstrate his love for his children.[2]

Essential oils have been used for therapeutic purposes for nearly 6,000 years. The ancient Chinese, Indians, Egyptians, Greeks, and Romans used them in cosmetics, perfumes, and drugs. Essential oils were also commonly used for spiritual, therapeutic, hygienic, and ritualistic purposes.

Essential oils are the regenerating, protective, and immune-strengthening properties of the plants. And since the human body chemistry is much like plant chemistry, the molecules in the oils mimic the molecules in the human body in repairing and strengthening itself. They can be antibacterial, antiviral, anti-infectious, anti-fungal, anti-inflammatory, analgesic, and they can provide emotional, physical, and spiritual benefits.

Most of us would agree that alternatives to Western Medicines at this time are important knowing that there is an increasing development of antibiotic resistance, overuse of drugs, dependency, and intolerances to pharmaceuticals. However, there are many who have similar reactions to essential oils and other plant medicines because of cheap extraction methods.

Quality does matter when it comes to essential oils! Because the effectiveness is based on the chemical constituents in the oil itself, the extraction method, indigenous environment, climate, season, time of day harvested, part of plant harvested, soil conditions, fertilizers, and more effect the outcome and ultimately the benefits to the body. Essential oils found in many stores and companies are often found to be adulterated in some way: additives, refinement, preservatives, dilutions (up to 90%) and/or solvent extracted. Even though the fragrance may be pleasant, the health benefits may be greatly reduced, and in some cases, toxic. Choosing high-quality, therapeutic-grade essential oils is important if you want superior results.

Many medical professionals are even coming forth one by one as they are introduced to the powerful benefits of essential oils, and are having phenomenal success with their uses, which is exciting to know they value something that is complementary to their practice.

Within the pages throughout this book you will find in each of The 7 Secrets, how essential oils, their purity and potency straight from nature, are capable of accelerating wellness in numerous ways through applications aromatically, topically, and/or internally (any or all of these). Most important, you will began to understand how nature is intended to support and strengthen your body, provide superior results to your healthcare needs, and you will become empowered to take more control of your health with the use of essential oils and an Eastern Medicine approach.

## CELLULAR HEALTH

Our cells are the fundamental units of life – the smallest components considered to be living organisms which make up your body's tissues and organs. Cells are constantly communicating with each other and responding to your environment and your body's needs. If your cells are deprived of vital nutrients and important dietary components, this can lead to low energy levels, emotional challenges, increased stress, disease, dysfunction, early aging, and a variety of poor health conditions. In other words, if your cells cannot operate efficiently, you will eventually experience diminished physical and emotional wellness.

The average adult has around 30 trillion cells within his or her body. Cells have three primary functions:

1) mitosis – to replicate on a regular basis
2) specialized function – as a nerve cell, muscle cell, blood cell, etc.
3) apoptosis – to self-destruct as needed on a regular basis

All of these functions rely on important dietary components, effective cleansing, adequate oxygen, and the proper tools to repair when damaged.

Two very important roles your cells play are in protecting your DNA from damage, and providing energy for everything your body requires. Within the cell is the mitochondria – the cellular engine – responsible for the energy of the cell and ultimately the energy of the body. The mitochondria relies on organic molecules that are derived from food sources: fats, carbohydrates, proteins, enzymes, and trace minerals. By keeping your cells well-nourished and supplied with the proper nutrients, you can keep your body well and functioning optimally too.

Your core focus within your lifestyle and habits – what you eat and drink, your activities, your environment – should be on keeping your cells healthy. If you really focus on your cells and supplying them with their needs, taste and bad habits become secondary to healthy lifestyle habits.

Here's an example:

Several years ago when my oldest grandson was only four years old, he came to spend the day with me. As we sat down for lunch, I cut up some carrots sticks and placed them on his plate. Immediately he looked up at me and said, "I don't want those, Nana. I don't like those." I tried to reason with him and explain that he needed to eat them because they were good for him, but found no success. Then the thought came to me that I expressed to him, "I think what you are telling me is that your tongue or taste buds don't want those, but did you know that your muscles and bones love carrots because they make you strong and run real fast?" Wow – that's all it took for him to gobble them all down!

Think cellular. That's where health begins. That's where your focus should be if you desire great health!

## HOW TO MAKE POSITIVE CHANGES IN YOUR LIFE

If you really want to change the outcome in your life, YOU CAN! Here's simply what it's going to take:

1) A HUGE DESIRE! You can't just hope for vitality and order in your body, or want it a little bit. It's got to be something you really, really yearn for. If you want to know the secrets of wellness and live the lifestyle of healthy, happy people, then you've got to want it badly enough to do whatever it takes to get just that. Commit right now to doing whatever it will take. It's worth it, and you can do it!

2) You've got to TRAIN YOUR MIND TO THINK DIFFERENTLY! If you don't like the space you are in, guess what? You've got to get OUT of it and into a new space! It's as simple as that. No more stopping at your old favorite stores, fast food favorites, ice cream parlors. I can hear it right now…yes, you've got to train your mind to think the way healthy, happy people do. Healthy, happy people realistically are not stopping at the same places you are, or they wouldn't be living the lifestyle they live. Does that make sense? And "as a man thinketh, so is he" applies here too.

If you are determined to eat well and build healthy habits while your thoughts are on being deprived of something more tasty and desirous, your body knows that! Your physical body will follow suit in what your mental body is telling you...so you must train your mind to THINK the way healthy, happy people do!

3) Next you've got to BE CHOOSY! Yes, healthy, happy people are choosy people. They understand that quality and content are more important than taste and cost...and that doesn't mean they have loads of money. Statistics show that you will spend 10 percent on prevention and 90 percent on the treatment of disease. Buying cheap food isn't cheap at all...it leads you on a road of disorder, dysfunction, and myriad disease treatments. That is what is costing you money! In the long run, you can avoid the high costs of treatments for the most part by being choosy. Choose quality and content over taste and cost! Be frank in turning down the plates of goodies and ignoring grocery store ads. Again, think cellularly and think to please your cells – that's what matters if you choose health.

4) EDUCATION is what this book is all about. Within these pages you will find many pieces of sensible information – and it will change your health, your weight, your energy, your mood, and your life IF YOU APPLY what you learn. I learned years ago in my study of world history, American history, and the slavery issue – FREEDOM WAS WON and achieved because of education! If you want the freedom from what ails you, then learn wellness, live wellness, and share wellness with others. This is a continual daily process, so keep learning and applying what you are learning each and every day. You will win!

5) Having a PERSONAL MENTOR to guide you is vital. I attribute my greatest success for making the needed changes necessary for my body to get well to having a mentor who guided me through the process. You will flounder on an unfamiliar path without someone who knows the way, goes the way, and shows you the way. I can provide that for you personally or match you with one of my professional team members. I am just being realistic when I say that you will absolutely need a mentor to guide you through the process of choosing a healthier path!

# NOURISH

# Chapter 1

# WHOLE FOODS

In my first career, I worked as a hairdresser. After working in the beauty shop for a few years, I became a stay-at-home mom with my first child and those who followed. However, I continued on with a few patrons coming to my home, and even several on a weekly basis for years. One particular woman came to see me one day each week for a matter for twelve to fifteen years. At a particular period of time, she began bringing her four-year old granddaughter, which was fine as I had children around her age to play with. But she, Angie, was an active child and often got into all kinds of mischief.

One particular day, after finishing up with the grandmother, I proceeded to check on the children and was horrified at what I found. It looked as if a tornado had gone through the family room…every puzzle piece was out of its box, every marble, every block, every toy and book was in disarray. Looking for the children, I found the bathroom in a similar fashion…soaps, cleansers, toilet paper, hair accessories were everywhere but where they belonged.

I turned to the grandmother and said that I could not deal with this any longer. There was always major clean up after Angie left, but this time was far worse than ever before. I had had it, and I couldn't do it anymore. Her grandmother responded that neither could her daughter! I got it! Grandmother was bringing this child each week to give mom a three-hour break – and I had to deal with the consequences!

I asked about her situation. Angie was hyper, hard to control, always making disasters and it was getting progressively harder to deal with her. So I asked the grandmother what her typical diet was, and her response was, "Nothing good!"

"Is her mother open to change?" I asked.

"She's open to anything that might work!" was the response.

"Anything?" I asked.

"Yes, anything!"

"Well," I said, "tell her to take her off of all white sugar, processed foods, milk products, and give her loads of fresh fruits and vegetables, whole grain cereals, and lean proteins." The grandmother said she would give her daughter that information and left.

It was two to three weeks before Angie returned, and I will never forget those moments when she came into the house, went straight to the toy cupboard, pulled down some books, went to the sofa, and began to read. They drugged her, I thought! I got the nerve to ask her grandmother, "What happened to Angie?"

"Her mother changed her diet as you suggested," was her response.

Wow! Over the next few weeks and months, I continued to marvel as I watched this little girl who had gone from Angie to Angel in such a short period of time. She was a changed little girl! She was sweet, content, and played happily without any type of hyperactivity or out-of-control behavior that was formerly her typical self. Eventually she started school, and I didn't see her for many years after that. I often thought of how this diet change saved her from being labeled in school as: ADD, ADHD, behavioral problems, lack of focus, always into mischief, emotional problems, poor grades, etc. Not only that, but she was a perfect candidate for behavioral problem medicines with all the side effects. Instead, her mother simply removed foods in her diet that were lacking nutrients and high in toxicity, and replaced them with fresh whole foods – full of nutrition, fiber, enzymes, antioxidants, and balance.

Several months back, I connected with Angie on Facebook and said, "Angie, I've told your story so many times over the past two years." Her response was, "Yes, my mother has told me that same story over and over as well." Well I'm not sure what her mother's story was exactly, but I do know that her little body was starving for nutrition and receiving just that changed her life and future, literally!

How many children do you know who are in the same type of situation as Angie?

## The Daily Basic 10

Most of us don't realize what constitutes a healthy diet and what we need on a daily basis. Here's what I refer to as The Daily Basic 10. The first three on the list are considered *macro*nutrients being a large portion of our diet. Then we have *micro*nutrients and although they have a minimal presence in the body, they are essential. Without them, our daily biological processes will lack proper function. Then of course we have water.

1) **Proteins** – building blocks, important for growth and repair of tissue
2) **Carbohydrates** – the body's source of fuel and energy
3) **Fats** – supports, protects, lubricates and insulates the body, vital for brain food
4) **Fiber** – a must for moving our food and waste through the intestines
5) **Vitamins** – for normal cell function, growth, development
6) **Minerals** – essential for bones and all human bodily functions
7) **Enzymes** – providing catalytic action aiding digestion
8) **Antioxidants** – protection for our cells from free radical damage
9) **Probiotics** – providing good intestinal floral to keep digestion in check
10) **Water** – essential for cleansing inside and out

Here's an interesting experience I had. A few years ago, I entered a home in preparation for teaching a class on nutrition, and as I began setting up for my presentation, the family was cleaning up dinner. First, I noticed the six-year-old who kept bouncing like a ball in excitement to show me his collection of artwork. Second, I noticed what the family dinner consisted of: cold cereal, milk, and chocolate-frosted-pudding-filled doughnuts for dessert. Let's take a look here and compare it to The Daily Basic 10:

- some protein (in milk)
- scads of carbohydrates (sugar, white flour, sugar, more sugar, and white flour galore)
- plenty of fats (in the doughnuts)

The meal was greatly deficient in fiber, vitamins, and minerals, basically no enzymes, antioxidants, probiotics, or water (and milk is not water). Yet this is typical for many individuals and families for breakfast and sometimes even dinner.

After the event, I learned from a close family friend that all four children in this family were some of the worse cases of ADD known in the neighborhood. Would one question why?

Let's take a look at each of The Daily Basic 10.

# Chapter 2

# PROTEIN

Protein is found throughout the body, our building blocks made from amino acids. Some amino acids are produced by the body, while others are "essential" and must come from our food sources. The body relies on having a good balance of these amino acids in order to transport nutrients, oxygen, and waste throughout the body as well as provide the structure, function, and regulation of cells, tissues, and organs.

Our western society, particularly the US and Canada, relies heavily on animals for our primary nutritional needs. Diets are typically full of beef, pork, poultry, eggs, cheese, and milk. Many of us have been raised with these foods as our traditional staples, but it's time we take a good look to understand what we are really eating.

What is wrong with a diet full of animal proteins? After all, we do need good protein and B vitamins. Milk and other dairy products contain high levels of calcium and fat, both of which are important for the development of young children. Plus, doctors tell us that we need milk to prevent osteoporosis (although there is significant controversy surrounding this).

Conventionally, it is common for animals (primarily cattle, pigs and chickens) to be given excessive amounts of antibiotics because they are living in cramped conditions, which limits physical activity and produces a toxic and diseased environment. It is also common for animals to receive regular doses of hormones of speed up the growing process. The hormones and antibiotics are not only present in the meat and dairy products you purchase from the regular grocery store, but they also can end up in the consumer...you! Is it any wonder that health problems seem to increase exponentially in those whose diets are full of meat and dairy?

As we take a look at popular diets, we see *The China Study* denoting that all animal foods—no matter the source—are responsible for modern ailments like heart disease, cancer, and more. Yet when we take a look at what Dr. Weston A Price's ten-year study concluded, we see it much differently.

## Doctor Westin A. Price Studies

Dr. Weston A. Price was a dentist in the 1930s who had a real interest in understanding why there were often such great variables in people's teeth. While some were notably perfect – little to no cavities, perfect jaw line without any crowding of teeth, there were others that had very inferior teeth (even when the parents' teeth were almost perfect). After much research, he decided that he and his wife would tour the world visiting indigenous cultures to see how their diets differed from the western diets and how this might influence the structure and health overall as well as the teeth.

This tour lasted over ten years of living with and studying the diets of many indigenous cultures around the world including those found in: New Zealand and other Polynesian islands, the Sudan tribes of Africa, the Aboriginals of Australia, American Indians from the mainland, Canada and Alaska, the Swiss, the Andes Mountain and Amazon Jungle Indians (from Peru and Bolivia), and more.

In the fifteen or more indigenous civilizations studied, there was a notable common thread. Even though the diets differed in each group, those who had superior physical and emotional health were those who ate their native whole foods diet – eating only the foods they grew or could find nearby, what they hunted or fished, or what they raised in their own vicinity. In these cultures:

- People ate mostly a plant-based diet that they either grew themselves, traded with neighbors, or purchased locally.
- Vegetables and fruits included: greens, sweet potatoes, bananas, berries, etc.

16

- Animals were wild caught, most were from the sea, and all others animals ate in the wild.
- Sea vegetables were important for vital nutrients.
- Grains and legumes were harder to grow and were rarely eaten among most of the tribes visited, but any present were in a whole-food form (not in flour and especially not refined).
- Foods were all nutrient dense – high in vitamins, minerals, and fiber
- Civilizations in the study consumed few milk products except in Switzerland and two African tribes, and all milk was completely raw.

In these indigenous civilizations, he found:

- Entire cultures with no tooth decay, crowded teeth, or misshapen dental arches

- These cultures also experienced no cancer, heart disease, diabetes, arthritis, hormonal problems, mental illness (Western diseases or disorders in general).

- More impressive than their physical strength, "was their character, their courage, honesty, dedication to family, they never stole and were completely trustworthy, they lived completely in the interest of others, there was no hunger and no crime."

- No processed foods were among the healthy tribes, yet once tribal members moved to cities and ate/adopted the processed/refined foods, not only did they develop notable tooth decay, missing teeth and jaw deformities, they also experienced infertility, miscarriages, and became susceptible to acute diseases: arthritis, cancer, heart disease, diabetes, weight gain, digestive disorders, and other chronic diseases. Plus "their behaviors changed, they experienced changes in brain functions, and immoral actions were accompanied by a lack of common sense."[3]

Physicians who interviewed the native people living on their indigenous diets testified that these people remained nearly or entirely free of all disease throughout their lives.

## Babies and Children in Dr. Price's Study

His study also included in-depth study of how these cultures produced healthy babies and children. This included:

- how couples prepared months before conception eating "sacred foods" (liver and more) given up from tribal members and saved for couples preparing to conceive.
- these cultures sacrificed these "sacred foods" for any pregnant mother to make sure she had proper nutrition.
- babies were nursed with no supplementation for the first eight to twelve months, and three to four years total.
- diets of toddlers were high in nutrition, and they were given only the foods their teeth could chew, food the adults ate.
- the cost for babies was nothing significant as it wasn't anything extra.

Contrast babies and children today. What are their first foods, the snacks they consume, when do they normally begin eating, and why? Might we wonder why we have the apparent childhood diseases, and why our "pre-school age children are the fastest growing age group being prescribed antidepressants"[4] simply because they are being deprived of the vital nutrition that would keep them well?

Next, we see *The Paleo Diet,* which greatly corresponds with Dr. Price's study in promoting:

- Vegetables and fruits in abundance – being a large part of one's diet, 75 percent or more
- Healthy fats from nuts, seeds, avocados, olive oil, coconut oil
- Lean grass-fed meats, eggs, fish for fat and protein sources
- Elimination of most grains, breads, flours and anything refined (sugar, flour, fats)

However, you do need to understand a huge issue pertaining to animal protein that is often missing in some of the studies or other information presented simply because of the time period written or lack of emphasis. Here it is:

Quality matters! All chicken is not equal – all fish is not equal – all beef is not equal either. Chicken, for example, from your mainstream grocery stores, fast-food places, and restaurants mostly come from commercial growers who are using antibiotics, vaccines, growth hormones, GMO corn/soy feed, crowded cages, and chemicals in the soaking process. This is going to constitute a completely different end product than chicken raised on an open range, organically grown grass-fed environment, which are minimally processed and without chemicals. The taste and flavor is notably different! And its ability to nourish or pollute your body based on which you choose is notably different as well. Think about it. You are actually eating the lifestyle of that animal – and guess what, that will influence your lifestyle as well. Eat a couch potato, and you become one too!

Additionally, your choices of meats can greatly differ in protein, fat, and omega content. See the following chart that compares wild game to feedlot (commercial grown) meats:

## COMPARISON OF:
# PROTEIN & FAT IN
# WILD GAME AND MODERN FEEDLOT MEATS
### (3.5 OUNCE PORTIONS)

| WILD GAME | GRAMS OF PROTEIN | GRAMS OF FAT |
|---|---|---|
| Goat | 20.6 | 3.8 |
| Rabbit | 21.0 | 5.0 |
| Deer | 21.0 | 4.0 |
| Bison | 21.7 | 1.9 |
| Elk | 22.8 | 0.9 |
| Turkey | 25.7 | 1.1 |
| Salmon (wild caught) | 23.4 | 4.3 |

The average fat content of this group of wild game is 2.8 grams, high in omega-3 fatty acids because of a diet in the wild that includes fresh greens, berries and seeds.

| MODERN FEEDLOT MEATS | GRAMS OF PROTEIN | GRAMS OF FAT |
|---|---|---|
| Prime Lamb Loin | 14.7 | 32.0 |
| Ham | 15.2 | 21.2 |
| Regular Hamburger | 17.9 | 21.2 |
| Choice Sirloin Steak | 16.9 | 26.7 |
| Pork Loin | 16.4 | 28.0 |
| Chicken Thigh | 21.0 | 13.0 |
| Salmon (farmed) | 22.1 | 12.3 |

Note the average fat content of the group of feedlot meats is 25 grams, being high in omega-6 fatty acids because of a grain fed diet (corn and soy to fatten) and being almost ten times higher in fat than the wild game.

In comparing the two, wild meat animals have a higher protein, lower fat content that is rich in omega-3 fats, while feedlot meats contain lower protein and a considerably higher unhealthy omega-6 fat content. Interesting![5]

Will your choices make a difference in how you feel and look? Is price the only thing to consider, or do you consider your cells' and body's needs when you make purchases?

Good health and natural weight balance is not an accident; it must be pursued with diligent effort. You can avoid what is harmful to your health and make better choices in animal proteins. Here are some suggestions:

- Consider raising your own animals – you are sure to eat them more sparingly
- Hunt for wildlife that has been eating in the open range without any hormones, antibiotics, or chemicals of any kind
- Shop smart for meats that are guaranteed to be from grass-fed, free-range animals which have not been given antibiotics or hormones. Again choose quality over cost.
- Choose wild-caught salmon or other ocean fish, and avoid any type of farmed fish.

Now let's take a look at plant proteins and what they also supply for us. Having a variety of proteins on a daily basis is a much healthier regimen than choosing all animal or all plant. Research tells us that because meat produces heat within the body in the digestive process, plant proteins should be eaten more when climate temperatures are hotter, so in other words, it is advantageous to eat more plant proteins in hotter weather and more animal proteins in cold weather.

Raw nuts and seeds, legumes and sprouts can be good sources of valuable protein when eaten within reason. Those organically grown without chemicals and pesticides are much preferred.

Almonds are one of nature's healthiest foods in a whole raw form. Here are some quick facts about raw almonds:

- healthy source of monounsaturated fats, which help reduce the risk of heart disease, also due to action of the vitamins E
- known to reduce LDL cholesterol – great for cardiovascular health
- high in magnesium, which improves the flow of blood, oxygen and nutrients throughout the body
- high in potassium for nerves, heart, and other muscles
- great source of protective antioxidants
- the only nut that is alkaline, which is why it is one of the better choices of nuts
- eating almonds with high glycemic foods will help reduce the glycemic index
- good for blood sugar control, thus a handful after a meal is a great dessert as well as very satisfying
- soaking almonds for 2-4 hours before eating (which can be kept in the refrigerator for several days) can greatly increase the nutrition content of the nut but also break down phytates that inhibit digestion

Ten almonds contain approximately:

- 2.5 grams protein
- 1 gram of dietary fiber
- 6 grams of fat

Even though this is a healthy source of protein, fat, and other important nutrients, if it were the sole dietary protein, the fat content would be way too high for the only protein consumed on a daily basis.

Most other nuts are of an acid content (see Acid to Alkaline chart) but are good when eaten raw for variety.

Legumes (beans, peas, lentils, peanuts) can also be a good source of protein. However because they (as well as grains, seeds, and nuts) contain phytates and enzyme inhibitors which can detract from their nutritive value, they should be soaked properly to maximize nutrient density by mitigating the effects of these anti-nutrients.

Beans vary from 14-17 grams per cup. The fat content is low, and the carbohydrate and fiber content are high. Cooked beans, peas, and lentils are great added to soups, salads, stir-fries, and are an excellent for making into hummus – a tasty spread or dip for crackers and vegetables. However, for best digestion make sure you include extra enzymes when eating any type of beans/legumes. A first step is having over half of your meal contents being raw greens or vegetables – a good hearty green salad is much preferred! Next, add a dietary enzyme complex for best digestion of nutrients and protein.

# Chapter 3

# CARBOHYDRATES

Carbohydrates are the body's chief source of energy. They are necessary for digestion and for the metabolizing of proteins and fats. We do need carbohydrates – but not from refined foods and in the quantities most often eaten.

From one who early on was a lover of breads, muffins, cakes, sweets – it's hard to believe I've come full circle in now promoting a diet that is mostly free of grains and bread products. I just feel better without them – my digestive system just works better, and the more I study these foods, I agree with the research that they are not in our best interest especially in the quantity most often consumed. As I first studied Dr. Price and found that very few of the healthy cultures he studied ate grains (possibly because they are harder to grow and harvest), this corresponded with much of the information available today. Let's see why.

Grains are the seeds of grasses which contain phytates or phytic acid which is a mineral blocker preventing the absorption of calcium magnesium, iron, and other minerals. Grains, soaked or sprouted, not only break down the phytic acid, but this increases the content of many important vitamins and minerals.

With considerable increase of grain consumption in the last one hundred-plus years, chronic disease rates have skyrocketed, fertility has fallen, and the average weight of the population has steadily risen. In addition, take into consideration the increased amounts of refined foods that have continually been introduced into the markets as fast foods in the past twenty to thirty years. This means more havoc in our systems, creating food sensitivities, weight gain, eating disorders, and more.

Studies show that eliminating most grains and breads can lower cholesterol, lower blood pressure, promote natural weight release, reduce inflammation, eliminate many skin disorders and digestive disorders, increase fertility and improve mood and energy levels.

Now most of you are thinking, "What, no pasta, breads, cereals, desserts or pastries! What is life without these foods?"

The more appropriate question is…what would my life really FEEL like without these foods?

## Eating Disorders

Each year, more than five million Americans are affected by serious and often life-threatening eating disorders that include anorexia, bulimia, compulsive eating, and binge-eating.

Although every age group and gender is affected, women in particular are targeted and suffer in many ways. It might surprise you to know that:

- Most women in the US and in other countries hate their figures.
- It is estimated that approximately 65 percent of Americans are overweight.
- Unhealthy weight gain due to poor diet and lack of exercise is responsible for over 300,000 deaths each year.[6]
- According to the American Society of Plastic and Reconstructive Surgeons (ASPS), more than 236,000 cosmetic procedures were performed on patients ages 19 and younger in 2012[7]
- Air brushing is a standard $60,000 computerized procedure for a magazine cover to remove blemishes, lift cheekbones, restructure the jaws and/or nose, increase the bust line, slim the hip line, and create the "perfect" woman who doesn't really exist (the woman on a magazine cover may only be a computerized constructed figure).
- Many teens and women perceive these figures and models as real and become dissatisfied with their own bodies, even if they are at a normal weight.
- Many, many women suffer with low self-esteem and depression. And although we may teach them principles of fulfilling the inward self, becoming who they are spiritually and mentally, and focusing

less on their outward appearance, the truth of the matter is that it is the nature of women (and all) to feel good physically and to look good physically not only to themselves – and especially themselves – but also to others.

Where does it start?

1) Diets from highly processed foods: advertised sales at the supermarket, fast food restaurants, and convenience stores.
2) Because these foods are depleted of vital nutrients, you crave more, eat more.
3) Overeating puts on extra pounds, and you feel emotionally stressed and depressed
4) This creates feelings of body hatred, needing to diet; however, a diet deprives you, and you end up putting on more weight
5) You go out in public and see too many obese people – then you see the billboards and magazines with cute, slender bodies, and you become dissatisfied with your own appearance. You try every fad diet (although none of them is effective in the long run), you become more depressed, which can spur you toward bulimia and anorexia, or binge-eating, compulsive eating, and obesity
6) It all goes downhill from there!

Most don't realize how bad processed foods really are and how a high-carb, high-grain diet is killing you emotionally, physically, spiritually, and mentally! What would your life really FEEL like without these foods?

You'd be surprised how easy it is to let go of something that is the culprit of so much havoc when you understand it!

# Chapter 4

# FATS AND FIBER

## Fats

Fat is the third major nutrient in your food along with proteins and carbohydrates. You need fat as a concentrated source of energy and protection for your brain and organs. Fats support, protect, lubricate, and insulate your body. They are vital for brain function and play a vital role in the health of your bones.

There are many misconceptions concerning fats making you fat. Remember the "no-fat", low-fat" craze back of the late 1980s? While fats were lowered or omitted in many products, sugars and additional calories were substituted. People interpreted that a product low in fat was good for them without thinking of what it contained instead of the fat, and actually more people gained weight during this craze. But there was something that was worse than that.

While the media continued to report fats as the culprit of obesity, they totally ignored the evidence that their subjects were carbo-loading on pasta, breads, cereals, muffins, doughnuts, and desserts, and failing to exercise. Because elevated insulin levels with this diet influences the biochemical processes that can lead to atherosclerotic plaque formation in the arteries, subjects experienced higher rates of heart disease than those who consumed more fat.[8]

Even though we do need omega-3, omega-6, and omega-9 fats, what most diets consume in fast foods is an overabundance of refined omega-6 Trans fats (coming from vegetable oils: corn, soy, safflower, cotton, canola, etc.) and are most often combined with refined sugars and flours. These three together – refined fats, sugars, and flours – are a major culprit for:

- most major diseases: heart disease, obesity, diabetes
- depression and other emotional dysfunction
- pain and inflammation

These Trans fats are what you really want to run from. They are artery-clogging fats produced by heating liquid vegetable oils in the presence of hydrogen to make them solid at room temperature – a process known as hydrogenation. Margarine, vegetable shortening, ice cream, processed cheese, potato chips, cookie dough, white breads, dinner rolls, snack foods, salad dressings are filled with Trans fats. Why? Trans fats in food products increase the shelf life.

Is your body and health considered in the creation of these foods? Do you need them or have to have them? You have a choice!

Quality and content is king! Healthy sources of fats include saturated fats (from butter, eggs), omega-3 polyunsaturated fats (salmon, tuna, other fish, flax, eggs), omega-9 monounsaturated fats (avocado, almonds, walnuts, other nuts, eggs).[9]

Be careful in heating oils and even nuts. We seem to be hooked on cooked, baked, and fried foods – though that may be necessary for meats. Keep the cooking of oils and roasted nuts to a bare minimum and use your fats raw as much as possible as a condiment: on salads, in dressings, in smoothies, etc. See Chapters 29 and 30 for recipes and suggestions for Salad Dressings that include good fats and essential oils.

Also, consider purchasing raw nut butters and raw tahini (sesame seed butter) over roasted. Roasted fats become rancid and toxic and need to be omitted as much as possible. And by the way, peanut butter not only contains aflatoxins – molds after being stored in warm, humid storage areas – which is a potent carcinogen, but it's not even a nut (but a legume) and doesn't fall into the healthy food category at all! Replacing it with raw almond butter and other raw nut butters is better for you.

# Fiber

Eating fiber is not an option in a healthy diet. It provides roughage or bulk for moving your food and waste through the intestines and keeping your system clean. However, often people think to purchase fiber as a separate item in supplement form or bran. That is simply not necessary. A diet full of fresh raw vegetables, fruits, nuts, whole grains or legumes provides ample natural fiber.

Dietary fiber is indigestible and is meant to be as such. Unlike other foods, it passes relatively intact through your stomach, small intestine and colon, and out of your body acting as a great housecleaner and sweeper for your system.

Two types of fiber:

1) Soluble fiber dissolves in water to form a gel-like material. It can help lower blood cholesterol and glucose levels. Soluble fiber is found in oats, peas, beans, apples, citrus fruits, carrots, barley and psyllium.

2) Insoluble fiber promotes the movement of material through your digestive system and increases stool bulk. Whole grains, nuts, beans and vegetables, such as cauliflower, green beans and potatoes, are good sources of insoluble fiber.

A high-fiber diet has many benefits, which include:

- Normalizing bowel movements by solidifying and increasing the weight and size of stool and decreasing your chance of constipation.
- Helps improve bowel health in lowering your risk for developing hemorrhoids, pouches in your colon, and other diseases that can develop in the colon.
- Lowers cholesterol levels by lowering low-density lipoprotein as well as reducing blood pressure and inflammation.
- Helps control blood sugar levels by slowing the absorption of sugar and improving blood sugar levels.
- Aids in achieving healthy weight because high-fiber foods generally require more chewing time, you feel fuller longer, and there is better cleansing and less stagnation present in the intestines and colon.[10]

How do you get more fiber in your diet? I hope you have a really good clue…loads of fresh raw vegetables and fruits! Eat them every chance you get. You will feel so much better with all the benefits they provide.

# Chapter 5

# VITAMINS AND MINERALS

Beside the *macro*nutrients proteins, carbohydrates, and fats, you also must have *micro*nutrients: vitamins, minerals, enzymes, and more. These are basically nonexistent in many diets but can no longer be ignored. Although they are present in smaller quantities than our *macro*nutrients, they too have a crucial part to play. They enable thousands of chemical actions that take place in the body every second of the day. Without them, basically you can't survive!

Vitamins are organic compounds found in both animals and vegetables. We find them in two forms: fat-soluble vitamins such as A, D, E, and K, which are stored in fat, and water-soluble vitamins such as B-complex and C, which are not stored in the body.

Minerals are found in inorganic compounds from our water and salt, as well as in organic compounds from our foods: meat, eggs, nuts, vegetable, fruits, and more. Black strap molasses, what's left over from refined sugar, is an excellent source of organic minerals. Some minerals, such as calcium, magnesium, potassium, phosphorus, and sodium are needed in higher quantities than our trace minerals such as zinc, iron, copper, chromium, selenium and others.

One of the best ways to increase your daily vitamin and mineral content is by choosing whole foods…everything whole as much as possible. And especially include more fresh raw vegetables, greens, and fruits in your diet. If today you wanted to make ONE BIG CHANGE in your health that would make the biggest difference, it would most likely be to include more fresh raw vegetables, green salads, and fruits in your diet – especially vegetables and greens. These all are needed not only for the vitamin and mineral content, but for the fiber, enzymes, reduced calories, water rich cleansing, antioxidants, and the alkalizing balance of your body.

Simply put, vitamins and minerals are necessary for energy production, and for the support and building of hormones, tissues, muscles, and bones. In addition to eating good whole foods, having a good balanced supplement is highly advantageous over purchasing supplements a la carte. In fact, purchasing a la carte is often times a waste of your money because the body is looking for balance, whole-food nutrition that is in a food form. If these essential nutrients are not consumed in balance, the effectiveness of any single nutrient is greatly reduced, if not nullified entirely. However, this doesn't mean there isn't ever a need for additional nutrients in higher quantities for target health, but to be effective, you still must start with a good balanced supplement to begin with.

In Chapters 16 and 17, we will go into this in more detail as we look at overall balanced, whole-food nutritional supplements and their delivery system.

## Alkaline and Acid Foods

All foods that we digest release an alkaline base (bicarbonate) or an acid into the blood and tissues of the body depending on the mineral compounds the food contains. Acidosis is the complete opposite of alkalosis.

There is plenty of research showing the link between acidic pH and cancer. Basically cancer thrives in an acidic environment and cannot survive in an alkaline environment. According to Keiichi Morishita in his book, *Hidden Truth of Cancer,* when your blood starts to become acidic, your body deposits acidic substances (usually toxins) into cells to allow the blood to remain slightly alkaline. This causes your cells to become more acidic and toxic, which results in a decrease of their oxygen levels and harms their DNA and respiratory enzymes.

Over time, he theorizes, these cells increase in acidity, and some die. These dead cells themselves turn into acids. However, some of these acidified cells may adapt in that environment. In other words, instead of dying – as normal cells do in an acid environment – some cells survive by becoming abnormal cells. "These abnormal cells are called malignant cells.

# Alkaline to Acid Chart

| Food Category | Most Acid | Acid | Lowest Acid | Lowest Alkaline | Alkaline | Most Alkaline |
|---|---|---|---|---|---|---|
| Sweeteners | NutraSweet Equal, Aspartame, Sweet n' Low | White Sugar, Brown Sugar | Processed Honey, Molasses | Raw Honey, Raw Sugar | Maple Syrup, Rice Syrup | Stevia |
| Fruits | Blueberries Cranberries Prunes | Sour Cherries, Rhubarb | Plums, Processed Fruit Juices | Oranges, Bananas, Cherries, Pineapple, Peaches, Avocados | Dates, Figs, Melons, Grapes, Papaya, Kiwi, Berries, Apples, Pears, Raisins | Lemons, Watermelon, Limes, Grapefruit, Mango, Papaya |
| Vegetables | | Potatoes (without skins) | Cooked Spinach, String Beans | Carrots, Tomatoes, Fresh Corn, Mushrooms, Cabbage, Potato Skins, Olives | Okra, Squash, Green Beans, Beets, Celery, Lettuce, Zucchini, Sweet Potato | Asparagus, Onions, Vegetable Juices, Parsley, Raw Spinach, Broccoli, Garlic |
| Beans Legumes | Chocolate | Pinto Beans, Navy Beans, Lima Beans | Kidney Beans | Peas, Soybeans, Tofu | Carob | |
| Nuts & Seeds | Peanuts, Walnuts | Pecans, Cashews | Pumpkin Seeds, Sunflower Seeds | Chestnuts | Almonds | |
| Oils | | | Corn Oil | Canola | Flax Seed | Olive Oil |
| Grains Cereals | Wheat, White Flour, Pastries, Pasta | White Rice, Corn, Buckwheat Oats, Rye | Sprouted Wheat Bread, Spelt, Brown Rice | Amaranth, Millett, Wild Rice, Quinoa | | |
| Meats | Beef, Pork, Shellfish | Turkey, Chicken, Lamb | Venison, Cold Water Fish | | | |
| Eggs Dairy | Cheese, Homogenized Milk, Ice Cream | Raw Milk | Eggs, Butter, Yogurt, Buttermilk, Cottage Cheese | Soy Cheese, Soy Milk, Goat Milk, Goat Cheese, Whey | Breast Milk | |
| Beverages | Beer, Soft Drinks | Coffee | Tea | Ginger Tea | Green Tea | Herb Teas, Lemon Water |

11

Malignant cells do not correspond with brain function nor with our own DNA memory code. Therefore, malignant cells grow indefinitely and without order. This is cancer."[12]

Actually, too much acidity in one's diet is an underlying factor in many degenerative diseases: diabetes, arthritis, heart disease, fibromyalgia, and more. But again, you can make a choice to be proactive and most likely avoid these degenerative diseases by taking action to make your body more alkaline.

Study the Acid to Alkaline chart above and you will see that the majority of foods consumed are acidic such as meat, grains, sugar, and milk. In fact, the typical American diet is all on the most acid column. If you want to change that and work to alkalize your system – you can do that simply by choosing to eat loads of fresh vegetables and fruits. That's what it's really going to take to get a neutral pH balance…and it's simpler than you think!

Tips that may help you:

- Eat raw vegetables or fruits with every eating interval…breakfast, lunch, dinner, and even at snack time, eat apples or celery with raw almond butter, for example. Fill up on your fresh raw produce first.

- Include more greens: add them to a smoothie in the morning (see recipes in Chapter 30), always include a green salad with lunch and dinner being the larger portion of your meal.

- When possible, choose alkaline sources over acids: almonds over other nuts; quinoa, amaranth, millet over other grains; stevia, pure maple syrup and honey over sugar; carob over chocolate; herbal teas over black tea or coffee.

- Lemons cannot be considered as base or alkaline until after digestion. Because of its sour taste no one will dispute that it actually contains acid. However, once a person absorbs the nutrients of lemon, the end product produces alkaline ash or residue. It oxidizes to form water, inorganic compound, and carbon dioxide after digestion that makes it alkaline as the end result. [13]

## What Might be Creating Food Sensitivities?

Have you ever stopped and wondered why so many individuals today have so many food sensitivities? Wheat, peanuts, soy, milk, nuts, and eggs – do you have any clue why?

Take a look at what is typical for commercial growing of most crops in the US:

1. Commercial farmers plant grains/seeds that are typically hybrids (cross-pollinated), GMO (Genetically Modified Organisms or better defined as 'God Move Over'), and Round-Up ready (grains infused with pesticides to repel insects).

2. Plants are grown with pesticides, chemical fertilizers, germicides, fungicides – all chemicals which are absorbed into the foods, plus they contaminate and deplete the soil of its vital nutrients.

3. Produce is harvested prematurely for transportation, and is often coated with waxes and colors, and irradiated to extend shelf life.

4. Grains are refined, bleached, and processed to remove fiber and fats (for a longer shelf life).

5. Foods are recreated with added trans fats (for increased shelf life), refined sugars, artificial colors, artificial flavorings, artificial sweeteners, enhancers, additives, preservatives – all in chemical form

6. Next they are overcooked: bottled or canned (laden with lead), and microwaved (which changes the molecular structure).

When these foods are introduced into your body, it cries out with "What the heck is this? I don't recognize it as a food – it has no nutrients, it's full of chemicals, the cell structure is foreign – I need tools to be able to function properly! I cannot use these!" Eventually the body gives up trying, it breaks down, and finally says "No more! I'm worn out! I'm done! I can't handle this anymore!"

Is it a wonder why there are so many food sensitivities? Leaky gut? Digestive dysfunction? Instead choose to eat and grow whole organic foods if at all possible!

## Do You Really Need Milk?

"It's not natural for humans to drink cow's milk. Human's milk is for humans. Cow's milk is for calves. You have no more need of cow's milk than you do rat's milk, horse's milk or elephant's milk. Cow's milk is a high fat fluid exquisitely designed to turn a 65 lb. baby calf into a 400 lb. cow. That's what cow's milk is for!" – Dr Michael Klaper, MD

"I no longer recommend dairy products after the age of 2 years. Other calcium sources offer many advantages that dairy products do not have." – Dr. Benjamin Spock

Here are some quick facts about milk:

- Today's dairy cows each produce about 100 pounds of milk per day—10 times more than cows living just a few decades ago. This is due to bovine growth hormones, unnatural diets, and being bred selectively for massive milk production.
- Unnaturally high milk production leads to mastitis, a painful bacterial infection causing a cow's udder to swell. Thus routine antibiotics and vaccines are administered to keep mastitis under control.
- Just as with humans, cows naturally only produce milk as a side effect of giving birth. Their milk is meant for their young. To keep the milk flowing, dairy farms artificially inseminate cows once a year. Their gestation period lasts nine months, so the majority of dairy cows' lives are spent pregnant. When a calf is born, he or she is removed from the mother—generally that same day—to make the mother's milk available for collection. Male offspring are often raised for veal, while females become the next generation of dairy cows. [14]

Growing evidence is showing that calcium in milk does not protect against osteoporosis. For example in a twelve-year Harvard study of 78,000 women, those who drank milk three times a day actually broke more bones than women who rarely drank milk. Similarly, a 1994 study in Sydney, Australia, showed that higher dairy product consumption was associated with increased fracture risk: those with the highest dairy consumption had double the risk of hip fracture compared to those with the lowest consumption. [15]

If you want milk on occasion, make the switch to milks made from coconut and almonds and eat a diet high in greens, vegetables, fruits, raw nuts and seeds to provide you with the calcium and other vitamins and minerals you need.

# Chapter 6

# ENZYMES, ANTIOXIDANTS, AND PROBIOTICS

Enzymes are complex molecules that enable thousands of essential biochemical reactions in the body. They aid digestion, break down toxins, strengthen the immune system, build protein into muscle, eliminate carbon dioxide from lungs, and reduce stress on the pancreas and other vital organs. In order to digest and assimilate the food we eat, we need enzymes. Without them, digestion is inhibited, undigested foods can ferment, create toxins, clog our intestines, produce inflammation, and result in a wide variety of illnesses, diseases, and premature aging.

There are different classes of enzymes. Metabolic Enzymes are produced by the body, and play a vital role in the functioning of virtually every system and organ within us. Digestive Enzymes, which are produced by the pancreas and other organs, break down the food we eat, enabling the body to get the benefit of the life-giving nutrients food offers.

Our body was NEVER meant to produce all the digestive enzymes needed for proper digestion. Nature packed raw, live foods with yet another class of enzymes – Food Enzymes – which happens to be many of the exact enzymes needed to let the body break down and digest the foods that contain them. Unfortunately, the natural enzymes from many fresh, raw foods are no longer alive when we finally eat them because: they are picked long before we eat them, they are cooked, have added chemical preservatives, irradiation, and/or other processing and preservation methods.

When we eat enzyme-deprived foods, our bodies "steal" metabolic enzymes from other parts of the body and put them to work digesting this food. Yet these enzymes are needed for the proper functioning of the body's organs and systems. The more we use them to digest food rather than let them be used as nature intended, and get our digestive enzymes from our raw foods, the more we jeopardize our health and vitality.

Increasing numbers of health professionals and nutritional scientists are becoming alarmingly aware that eating enzyme-depleted foods is a prime cause of illness, degenerative diseases, and premature aging. So where do we turn?

Eating a diet of raw, live, organic foods will supply us with most of the enzymes needed for easy and complete digestion of those foods. Realistically, however, after years and years of depriving our bodies of the natural enzymes and robbing them from other body parts for our digestion, we often have to rely on additional enzyme supplements. I have personally found phenomenal benefits from certain enzyme supplements in breaking down matter in the intestines and undigested proteins in the blood. We need enzymes.

Eating lots of raw foods will help increase your enzymes immensely – and better yet, will prevent the deprivation to begin with! Again, another reason to reach for more fresh raw vegetables, greens, fruits, nuts, sprouts, and any fresh live foods!

# ANTIOXIDANTS

Let's first address free radicals and how they are damaging to the human body, and how antioxidant nutrients help protect the body against free radical damage.

The human body is composed of many different types of cells. Cells are composed of many different types of molecules. Molecules consist of one or more atoms of one or more elements joined by chemical bonds. Normally, bonds don't split in a way that leaves a molecule with an odd, unpaired electron. But when weak bonds split, free radicals are formed. Free radicals are very unstable and react quickly with other compounds, trying to capture the needed electron to gain stability. Generally, free radicals attack the nearest stable molecule, "stealing" its electron. When the "attacked" molecule loses its electron, it becomes a free radical itself, beginning a chain reaction. Once the process is started, it can cascade, finally resulting in the disruption of a living cell.

Some free radicals arise normally during metabolism. Sometimes the body's immune system's cells purposefully create them to neutralize viruses and bacteria. However, environmental factors such as pollution, radiation, cigarette smoke, chemicals, and herbicides can also create free radicals.

Normally, the body can handle free radicals, but if antioxidants are unavailable, or if the free-radical production becomes excessive, damage can occur. Of particular importance is that free radical damage accumulates with age.

Antioxidants neutralize free radicals by donating one of their own electrons, ending the electron "stealing" reaction. The antioxidant nutrients themselves don't become free radicals by donating an electron because they are stable in either form. They act as scavengers, helping to prevent cell and tissue damage that could lead to cellular damage and disease.

Vitamins E and C offer antioxidant protection:

- Vitamin E may protect against cardiovascular disease by defending against LDL oxidation and artery-clogging plaque formation
- Many studies have correlated high vitamin C intakes with low rates of cancer, particularly cancers of the mouth, larynx, and esophagus.

Look at the ORAC (Oxygen Radical Absorbance Capacity) rating antioxidant levels of different foods, and see what you will find.

First, notice that clove essential oil is "off the chart" when it comes to antioxidant levels, and is something that you would benefit from in taking on a daily basis – I do for sure. Making sure your essential oil is recommended for internal use, just two drops daily under your tongue is highly beneficial to increase your anti-oxidant levels.

Fresh fruits and vegetables, though not as high individually, will accumulatively also provide great antioxidants that can help protect your body from free-radical damage. Hey – we might get this yet – just one more reason to be including 6-8 servings of fresh raw vegetables and fruits in your diet each and every day!

Yahoo for more fruits and vegetables for you!

| | ORAC |
|---|---|
| Clove essential oil | 1,078,700 |
| Cloves, ground | 314,446 |
| Cinnamon, ground | 267,536 |
| Oregano, dried | 200,129 |
| Tumeric, ground | 159,277 |
| Acai berry, freeze-dried | 102,700 |
| Wild Crafted Siberian Chaga | 52,452 |
| Small red beans | 13,727 |
| Blueberries | 2,400 |
| Cranberries | 1,750 |
| Kale | 1,770 |
| Broccoli | 890 |
| Orange | 750 |
| Apple | 218 |

16

## PROBIOTICS

Probiotics are live microorganisms or friendly bacteria cultures shown to enhance your entire digestive system and are critical to your overall health.

Your body contains billions of beneficial bacteria and microorganisms that assist the body in improving digestive efficiency. The lack of proper nutrients in the diet, the use of antibiotics, extended illness and aging can deplete healthy bacteria from your gut faster than it can be replenished. And without enough friendly flora, there are myriad issues that can occur in addition to many digestive dysfunctions.

It makes sense to include friendly flora foods in your diet on a daily basis. Here are some great suggestions:

- Yogurt – I prefer coconut milk yogurt, unsweetened vanilla.
- Coconut water kefir – you can even go online and make this easily yourself for a fraction of the cost – very healthy for you!
- Raw sauerkraut – another item that can be simply made and kept alive.
- Bragg organic apple cider vinegar. Great for restoring the pH balance in your body, it creates an alkalizing environment and encourages beneficial bacteria to grow by crowding out bad bacteria and aiding digestion. You can drink a mixture of two tablespoons apple cider vinegar mixed with 8 oz. of water. Do NOT add a sweetener because sugar will feed the yeast. [17]
- A good live prebiotic and probiotic supplement with a delivery system that will carry it all the way to the small intestines is optimal.

# Chapter 7

# WATER

Note that the first 9 of The Daily Basic 10 are foods providing tools to strengthen and support, while the last is water – essential for cleansing your body inside and out.

Water will be discussed in detail in the CLEANSE section, however, let's get a few facts straight here first.

IF IT'S NOT WATER, IT'S NOT WATER!

Soft drinks, Gatorade, sport drinks, energy drinks, alcohol, coffee, black tea, conventional milk, and fruit juices are not water. They can contain from 85-98 percent water, but the body does not see them as water, and here's why:

1. These items contain chemicals, additives, stimulants, sugars, and/or have been processed to the point of polluting the body. So whereas, water is a cleansing agent, these (for the most part) do just the opposite – they pollute and create toxicity.
2. Most of these drinks are surprisingly dehydrators and de-energizers. That's why one can go into a convenience store and buy 48 oz drinks on a continual basis because they are dehydrating, they do not hydrate the cells as water does.
3. These are all acid drinks, unlike water, which is a neutral ph. These acidic drinks can be the cause of osteoporosis, bone spurs, cancer, kidney stones, and a multitude of other diseases simply because they are acidic. Drinks that are alkaline are herbal teas and freshly made vegetable or fruit juices.

Your body needs water – good pure water:

- Vital for chemical reactions in digestion and metabolism
- Vital for cleansing the system of toxins
- Carries nutrients and oxygen to cells through blood
- Cools body through perspiration, and sweating is important for cleansing
- Lubricates the joints
- Needed for lungs to take in oxygen and excrete carbon dioxide
- Helps shed pounds and ultimately the best for healthy weight release
- Hydrated skin slows down aging process

I come across so many people who will say they drink a lot of water, when in reality they don't know how much a lot is. In a world where we are constantly bombarded with food, drink, and environmental toxicity, your body requires a minimum of approximately one-half of your body's weight in ounces daily. So if you weigh 150 pounds, you need to drink a minimum of 75oz of water each and every day, which is over two quarts.

However, if you:

- want to shed pounds
- live in a hot climate
- are experiencing illnesses consistently
- work out regularly
- are nursing a baby

you will best benefit by doubling that amount of water – or get your body's weight in ounces of water daily. Again, that's just water. If you are drinking other drinks in addition to this, those don't count. Remember, water is a vital component for optimum health for cleansing of your body inside and out.

# Chapter 8

# YOUR CHOICES OF FOODS

So would you like to know the secret on how whole foods can really create a whole new you? This understanding and visual can be life changing for you. It was for me!

Insulin and glucagon are both hormones produced in the pancreas that regulate levels of blood sugar (glucose) in your body. Your body produces glucose from the foods you eat, which is what fuels you. Insulin and glucagon are hormone partners working to keep your blood sugar levels in check, being the yin and yang of blood glucose maintenance. They are equally important in managing important bodily functions. [18]

Insulin is secreted by the beta cells in your pancreas when your blood sugar levels are high. It is designed to store the excess energy as fat. Eating a meal that is rich in refined carbohydrates that are high glycemic can cause your blood sugar levels to skyrocket, and your body to store more fat. [19] However, the greater concern than storing excess fat is that in eating an overabundance of these types of carbs, your pancreas goes into overtime producing insulin, and because of this, insulin can take too much glucose out of your blood. The result leaves you now in a state of low blood sugar…and you begin craving more carbs!! This cycle from high blood sugar to low blood sugar in a short period of time is a typical response with a diet of high-carb abundance, which not only keeps your blood sugar unstable, causes the formation of excess body fat, and is the culprit for most major dysfunction and disease.

Glucagon, on the other hand, is secreted by the alpha cells of your pancreas when blood sugar is low. This happens between meals, when exercising, but also with the right choice of foods. Fresh produce, balanced proteins, and complex carbohydrates will minimize insulin spikes, help keep your blood sugar in balance, increase glucagon, and promote fat burning naturally. Since glucagon causes the liver to release stored energy, with the choice of these foods, you ultimately feel more energetic and desire to be more active instead of sedentary.

Simply put, insulin and glucagon work in balance – as insulin increases, glucagon decreases, and visa-versa. Insulin promotes storing of energy while glucagon promotes the release of stored energy, both glucose and fatty acids.[20] Keep in mind that the pancreas is producing only one or the other at a time.

See the adjacent chart to understand this more simply:

The secret to all of this is that YOU have so much more control over which one is being produced more abundantly, how you store fat or burn fat, and whether your body responds with order or disorder. This is ultimately based on YOUR CHOICES OF FOODS. All you have to do is what we have been learning all along – choose whole foods based on nutrition, content and quality, NOT according to sales, your taste buds, the price, or calorie content!

One bonus secret…

If you want to accelerate the benefits, get faster results more effectively, then consider adding pure therapeutic essential oils – that are guaranteed safe for internal use to the foods that you eat and you can find these internal benefits:

- cleansing organs
- improving digestion
- stimulating your metabolism
- creating internal organ support and function
- increasing antioxidants
- building immunity
- raising your energy levels
- plus they add yummy flavors to your foods!

You can add essential oils to your water, your smoothie, salad dressings, dips, salsa, snack bars, frozen desserts, stir-fries, marinades, soups, yogurt…you name it! The ideas are endless!

# INSULIN & GLUCAGON

| FOR INCREASED INSULIN | FOR INCREASED GLUCAGON |
|---|---|
| **DIET RICH IN:**<br>• processed sugars<br>• white flour, high carbs<br>• ready-made prepared foods | **DIET RICH IN:**<br>• fresh vegetables & fruits<br>• lean animal proteins, raw nuts, plant proteins<br>• limited whole grains/ grain products |
| High in Carbs (sugars, flours)<br>High in Salt<br>High in Fats<br>High in Animal Proteins<br>Low in Fiber<br>Low in Enzymes for digestion<br>Low in Vitamins & Minerals<br>Low in Antioxidants | High in Fiber<br>High in Vitamins & Minerals<br>High in Enzymes for digestion<br>Balanced Complex Carbs<br>Balanced Proteins<br>Good Source of Antioxidants<br>Low in Salt<br>Low in Fats |
| **FAT GAIN/STORING MODE -**<br>Overweight or obese | **FAT BURNING MODE -**<br>Natural weight release/management |
| These foods clog, pollute, de-energize, are void of nutrition, and create DISORDER! | These foods cleanse, energize, support, strengthen, nourish, are full of nutrition, and promote ORDER! |
| Influences major diseases such as diabetes, heart disease, cancer | Influences good energy, emotional health, less disease/disorder |

See Chapter 29 and 30 for Creating Meal Plans as well as many tasty wellness recipes.

Healthy Happy People know the importance of a foundational diet consisting of good whole foods because you feel better, look better, and have more energy! And essential oils just increase the benefits!

## GOALS AND SUGGESTIONS

1) The next time you look at food and hear yourself say, "I really want this" or "I don't like this", what body part is speaking? Do you allow your taste buds to make ALL the decisions for your brain, organs, muscles, bones, blood, nerves, emotional health, physical health, and mental health? If you were to make all your food intake decisions according to ALL your body parts and functions, or according to the real "I", would your diet be totally different? These body parts love wholesome foods simply because they give them the ability to work in order, not disorder! So ask your brain, other organs, etc., before you make decisions in eating – and make it a conscious decision based on your needs, not wants.

2) Think about where you normally shop. Does your particular grocery store support healthy lifestyle habits? If you are to consider a lifestyle change, consider a new healthier market to do your shopping at too. This will make your transition much easier!

3) Think about the people within your reach. How many of them would benefit from learning this information? Call up a friend or family member today and share two things that have been most impactful for you. Invite them to come along with you, learn with you, and be your workout partner in wellness.

# CLEANSE

# Chapter 9

# REMOVING TOXICITY

Jenni is actually my daughter's friend, but I had the privilege of introducing Jenni to essential oils and have enjoyed getting to know her and her family. Sometime after that, Jenni went to the hospital for some minor female surgery and after coming home, five days later was taken back to the hospital with excruciating stomach pains only to find out she had c-diff (clostridium difficile). This situation is typically antibiotic induced and can also be highly contagious. Even though this is a bacteria always present in our gut, it normally has no ability to replicate unless an antibiotic wipes out the bad as well as the good intestinal flora, which can allow it to flourish dangerously enough to be life threatening.

After ten days of being in the hospital, Jenni did not improve. Her doctor came in early one Sunday morning and told her that they had done all they could for her, her organs were shutting down, she was dying, and she might consider preparing her family for the news. She thought and then sent me a text after four o'clock that Sunday morning. I ignored it and kept sleeping until I received another then another and finally decided to find out who might be so persistent. Jenni's text stated that she was dying while suffering from c-diff over the last ten days. She sent a photo of the toilet showing and told me: "I'm peeing black". She asked if I could help her, if I had any recommendations for her, and if I would be willing to come in and bring her some oils and perform an essential oil technique. I consented. At once I got to work doing some research, making preparations, and headed to the hospital. On the way, I got a call from my husband begging and pleading me not to go due to the risk for myself and possibly my family. I went anyway.

Jenni was down to 97 pounds at this point and was emotional as I went into her hospital room. Because of the risk of her condition, I was specifically told that anything that went in would not come back out…so upon going in I followed the request to cover myself with gloves, robe, and booties, knowing that any items brought in would have to be in containers to be disposed of. I basically did three things for her:

I gave her a large green smoothie that I had prepared for her full of fresh greens, fruits, and vegetables, nutritional additives and several essential oils. Later she told me that is was the first thing she was fully able to keep down her. She knew this was part of her healing, but it was very nasty! I don't remember what all I put in it.

I brought her a bottle of lemon essential oil suggesting that she literally drink it…putting several drops in her water throughout the day to cleanse out her internal organs as her urine was septic. Then I gave her the essential oil technique and application on her spine and feet. This was the first time I had given the technique with latex gloves on my hands.

The following day I called and texted Jenni with no response; the next day as well, with still no response. Finally I called my daughter, who said, "Mom, she came home yesterday!"

Wow! Jenni at that point was not well by any means, but her urine was clear and no longer septic, and she was feeling much stronger. She felt like she would get better care at home where she continued to regain her strength. Today, Jenni is vibrant, full of life and energy, and has a determined conviction to share the benefits of pure therapeutic grade essential oils with everyone around her.

Sometime later, I listened to a radio interview where Jenni was asked about this experience, and the big question was, "What did the doctor say about this? The fact that you were ready to go home about thirty-six hours after he said to call your family because you were about to die. What did he say?"

She said, "His response was quite different than I had expected. When he asked me what I had done, and I told him it was essential oils, his response was that they were dangerous and they could hurt me."

While I am grateful for the medical system being in place for emergencies, it's evident that there are often times when professionals know they have done all they can, and there are other options that can be more effective. Jenni's education and strong will to get better played a big role in her recovery. The essential oils provided the necessary cleansing action and support she needed, neurologically and physically, to bring order back to her body on a cellular level. In addition, she also added probiotics and other supplements for accelerating the process. Essential oils and other items from nature were the means for bringing life back to her body and allowing Jenni to continue to mother her four beautiful children.

My own initial experience verified this. With the presence of high levels of toxic metals and pharmaceuticals, I was experiencing many emotional and physical problems. I went through several rigorous cleanses in my first two months: lemon water cleanse, heavy metal cleanse, juice fasting, and colonics (to cleanse my colon rectally), and my body felt totally different (I knew nothing about essential oils back then). I had a great amount of energy, I could think, focus, and I felt great!

Remember, almost all dysfunction, disorder, and disease can actually be pointed to two main issues: 1) lack of nutrition and 2) too much toxicity. Any toxicity in the body can accumulate in the joints, organs, cells, and tissues creating inflammation, pain, and dysfunction.

What can create toxicity in the body?

- refined foods
- processed meats and cheeses
- chemical additives, preservatives, artificial colors and sweeteners
- soft drinks, sport drinks, energy drinks
- alcohol
- pasteurized/homogenized milk products
- pesticides and chemical cleaning products
- body care, hair care, skin care, nail care, sunscreens
- environmental toxicity
- pharmaceuticals
- plastic bags and bottles – absorb into your food and water
- microwave cooking your foods

We are bombarded with an enormous amount of these toxic substances on a daily basis. If your blood and urine were tested, most likely you would find hundreds of toxins derived from many of the above sources. One huge area of concern that may surprise you is that many women use up to 50 different substances on a daily basis (body care, skin care, hair care, perfumes, nail care, hand sanitizers, cleaning products, etc.) most of which contain toxic ingredients. And that is just one area on the list of things that you may encounter during your day. Add them all together and yes, there is toxicity in your body that needs regular cleansing, not just once a year like you do your spring cleaning, but on a daily basis. Cleansing regularly keeps your channels clear, free from buildup, and allows your body to function much more efficiently.

# Chapter 10

# SUBSTANCES THAT CAN CREATE TOXICITY

## Refined Foods

White sugar is pro-inflammatory, increases your appetite, stimulates weight gain, depletes your body of vitamins and minerals, promotes wrinkles, causes joint degeneration, promotes behavioral disorders, and is more addicting than cocaine! [21]

In addition, sugar irritates the linings of the stomach and intestine, lowers the hydrochloric acid content of the stomach, creates low stomach acidity, creates obesity, accelerates the growth of cancer, responsible for creating conditions as asthma, hay fever, eczema, hives, migraine or nervous headache, various food allergies stomach and bowel disorders, heart disease, hardening of the arteries, high blood pressure. [22]

"The definition of a food is, 'That which sustains life and promotes growth.' Sugar refined to the state of being a pure chemical or drug has been found to shorten life and stop growth. Therefore sugar can't be called a food. Like alcohol, sugar furnishes only calories to the body. A drug is defined as 'any substance used as a chemical ingredient in the arts.' Pharmacists agree that sugar meets the requirements of this definition of a drug." [23]

Studies show that children and adults can get up to 70 teaspoons of sugar per day in the foods they eat. [24] Did we understand that sugar meets the definition of a drug? And we seem to just overlook this?

High Fructose Corn Syrup (HFCS) is extremely toxic to your liver, causes blood sugar imbalances, increases chance for inflammation, and stimulates weight gain and stress.

On top of this, it's more addicting than refined sugar.

Partially Hydrogenated Oils (Trans fats) are found in thousands of processed foods to increase shelf life. Trans fat are proven to cause heart disease, increased inflammation, decrease immune system, increase your risk for arthritis, cancer, learning disabilities, diabetes, elevated blood pressure, heart disease, obesity, osteoporosis, and more.

Processed foods are NOT CHEAP when you consider the disorder and disease they create! Learn to avoid them like the plague…or reap the consequences like the plague!

## Processed Meats and Cheeses

As noted in Chapter 1, choosing quality meats from grass-fed free range animals is imperative. Mainstream market meats are raised with feed containing pesticides and other chemicals, are administered vaccines, hormones and antibiotics, often contain infectious parasites and that's just the beginning.

Processed meats contain nitrates and nitrites, which act as preservatives, colorings and flavorings, have been found to cause cancer and tumors in test animals. Plus they can contain a variety of animal parts such as "ground-up stomach, snout, intestines, spleens, edible fat, and even lips." [25]

Avoid ALL pork, shellfish, crustaceans, and catfish. Pigs are some of the filthiest animals, and their diet isn't any better. Shellfish, crustaceans, and catfish are ocean or lake bottom-feeders, sustaining themselves on fish waste and toxic waste. Remember what it eats, you eat too…and you won't want to eat what any of these have eaten!

To add to the toxicity, there are many refined soy meat substitutes that are anything but healthy because they are all highly refined. Unless it's organic, you can safely assume ALL processed soy milks, protein powder, tofu, soy burgers, soy ice cream, soy cheese and other soy junk foods are GMO products. If you choose any soy at all, make sure it is organic in one of these fermented forms: tempeh, miso, natto and soybean sprouts.

## Chemical Additives, Preservatives, Artificial Colors and Sweeteners

Monosodium glutamate is used in many foods to enhance taste, and has been associated with reduced fertility, migraine headaches, obesity, and other serious disorders.

Some of the worst of our chemical offenders are artificial sweeteners, sold to the American people as no-calorie, sugar-free products. Artificial sweeteners are harmful chemicals that can never have anything positive over sugar. They are addicting, noted for causing cancer, neurological problems, migraine headaches, dizziness, weight gain, increased appetite, bloating, rashes, hallucinations, brain seizures, and heart disease.

Artificial colors and other foods additives are known to contribute to behavioral problems, learning problems, emotional problems, hormonal dysfunction, allergic reactions, and cancer. In short, they cause negative changes in brain chemistry. [26]

If you want to avoid the side effects of these chemicals, then again, avoid them like the plague…or reap the consequences like the plague!

## Drinks

Why have we come so far to ignore the pollutions coming from the myriad of drinks available today? It's amazing to see our "eat, drink, and be merry" world dumbfounded when all of a sudden faced with a life-threatening disease…whereas people have "truly earned it" by their choices! This doesn't have to be you – you can choose differently especially when it comes to what you drink.

Instead, "eat, drink, and be wary" because not only are soft drinks, sport drinks, energy drinks filled with many chemical additives, preservatives, artificial colors, and artificial sweeteners that are toxic pollutants in your body (as stated above), they are acidic, they are dehydrators, and they contain stimulants that create addictions.

Have you heard of 4-Mel, also a popular carcinogenic additive in soft drinks? "The National Toxicity Program found 'clear evidence' of 4-Mel toxicity in sodas and linked 4-Mel to infertility, thyroid dysfunction and liver and lung cancer. After the report by National Toxicity Program about 4-

Mel toxicity, the State of California added 4-Mel to the list of chemicals linked to cancer.

"According to NTP, nine out of ten samples of Coke products purchased outside California had little or no trace of 4-Mel, whereas, 10 of 10 samples of Pepsi products purchased nationwide contained levels of 4-Mel that were about four to eight times higher than the safety levels set by California." [27]

Caffeine is a dehydrator that depletes your body of bonded magnesium, zinc and calcium as well as sodium, electrolyte and water. It is connected to high blood pressure, high cholesterol levels, malnutrition, birth defects, breast lumps, irregular heartbeat, and cancer. Hum, and people think it's okay to drink this stuff?

And what about energy drinks? In 2006, about 500 new energy drinks were introduced into the market. Again one of biggest concerns is caffeine. "Not all caffeinated drinks are created equal; the quantity of caffeine varies greatly from product to product. To put this into perspective, consider that most cola soft drinks have from 22 to 55 milligrams (mg) of caffeine, compared to a common cup of tea that varies from 26 to 47 mg. Coffee may have from 57 mg for a cup of instant to 180 mg for a cup of brewed. By comparison, energy drinks may have from 80 to 500 mg of caffeine in one can."[28]

Alcohol, beer and such are more potent toxic beverages that also need to be avoided. For something to be the cause of so many deaths, you'd think more than, "Don't drink and drive" one might post a more sensible statement that says, "Don't drink at all!"

Drinking alcohol disrupts brain function, interferes with communication, mood, behavior, physical coordination, and being able to think clearly. It stresses the heart, creating risks for stroke, high blood pressure, arrhythmias – irregular heartbeat, and heart disease. It damages the liver and pancreas, and challenges the immune system. Plus you are at higher risk for cancer: mouth, esophagus, throat, liver, and breast.[29] Where are you mentally when you drink even on occasion if you are putting yourself at these kinds of risks?

Don't be deceived into thinking that drinking any liquid is like drinking water. Water is a cleanser. All of these other drinks are toxic pollutants to your body! AVOID THEM and drink good pure water instead (with just a drop or two of your favorite citrus essential oil, coming up soon).

## Pesticides and Chemical Cleaning Products

All of these products, in a nutshell, have one goal in mind: to KILL microbes, pests, and/or pathogens. And if these products are meant to KILL…what might they be doing to you? Even more important, what might they be doing to children who are much smaller – an eighth, quarter or half your size?

The Food Quality Protection Act (FQPA) was the first law to acknowledge that infants and children need extra protection against pesticide exposures. "A toxin has much more devastating effects on a developing nervous system. The child's brain, because it is still growing, is much more vulnerable than an adult's brain," says Herbert Needleman, M.D., a professor of pediatrics at the University of Pittsburgh Medical School. "And because children lay on floors and on the ground, put their hands in their mouths, and eat more fruits and vegetables per pound of body weight, they receive a greater overall exposure to pesticides." [30]

An unacceptable amount of chemicals are saturating the environment, and it is affecting you and all of us more than you know. A documentary called *Unacceptable Levels* was recently produced that reveals how all these chemicals are truly affecting us:

- Autism now affects 1 in 50 children
- Cancer is the leading cause of death (after accidents) in children younger than 15 years in the US

In the last twenty years, the rates of asthma, allergies, and ADHD are on the rise:

- 400% increase in allergies
- 300% increase in asthma
- 400% increase in ADHD

- $2.6 trillion of the GDP is spent on treating disease every year.[31]

Almost all of our consumer products are made up of dangerous chemicals that do affect us negatively: pesticides and other chemicals in our foods, cleaning products, detergents, air fresheners, more. We will discuss this more in detail in Chapters 24-25.

# Body Care, Hair Care, Skin Care, Nail Care, Sunscreens

Your skin is the largest organ of your body. It provides protection for your structure and organs and is made up of several different components, including protein, water, lipids, and different minerals. How well do you care for it?

The skin care and cosmetic industry is unregulated, and sometimes the ingredients being used have not even been tested to ensure safety. Since your skin readily absorbs the products you use, it is super important to be aware of the possible dangers of certain ingredients that could harm your skin and body. What you use on your body is another important choice between nourishing or damaging your skin.

According to www.ewg.org (Environmental Working Group):

- More than one-third of all personal care products contain at least one ingredient linked to cancer.
- 57 percent of all products contain "penetration enhancer" chemicals that can drive other ingredients faster and deeper into the skin to the blood vessels below.
- 79 percent of all products contain ingredients that may contain harmful impurities like known human carcinogens, according to FDA or industry reviews. Impurities are legal and unrestricted for the personal care product industry. [32]

There are all kinds of products available out there. They do affect you one way or another, so be choosy! See Chapter 26 as we visit this entire topic more in depth.

## Environmental Toxicity

Each day, you are potentially exposed to many different kinds of toxicity found the air and environment:

- tobacco smoke
- chemical cleaners
- paint and lacquer, etc.
- pet dander
- mold, mildew
- dust and microbes
- airborne pathogens

It takes a conscious and consistent effort to avoid these substances, keep the air clean and your lungs free from toxicity.

## Pharmaceuticals

Pharmaceuticals are usually derived from chemical constituents created in laboratories. Because of their chemical nature, drug toxicity is common and can cause such symptoms as mental disorientation, dizziness, memory loss, fainting, blurred vision, and falling. Extended use of drugs, high doses of medications, body resistance to certain drugs, or a person's inability to metabolize a drug can all be reasons for drug toxicity which can accumulate and stress the organs of the body especially the liver and kidneys. Children and older people are naturally at a higher risk for drug toxicity. [33]

In Chapters 18-21, we will discuss this further and find natural solutions coming from essential oils and herbs, which most often are far superior without the side effects or toxicity levels attached.

## Plastic Bags

We live in a world full of plastic – yet another toxic substance you are exposed to on a daily basis. All plastic is made from chemicals, including BPA and DEHA, both are potentially harmful. Grocery bags are made from high or low density polyethylene and when storing foods in these bags, chemicals can leach into the food and then be ingested. Plastic bags, plastic wrap, plastic water bottles are all of concern, individually and collectively – just think of all that you might be using regularly. Over time these chemicals can be linked to genetic damage, chromosomal errors, tissue changes, miscarriage, birth defects, early onset of puberty, and hormonal changes. Children can particularly be affected by chemicals in plastic with a weakened immune system, hormonal disturbances, and behavioral problems.[34]

What's the solution? Here are some ideas:

- use paper or cloth bags when you shop
- remove all produce from plastics and place in large containers lined with cloth or paper towels (most produce can be washed and stored directly in your refrigerator fruit and vegetable bins: apples, tomatoes, peppers, carrots, etc. don't need to be bagged at all)
- use glass water bottles (with outside rubber protection)
- replace all your plastic containers and bowls with glass containers and glass bowls
- store refrigerated items in small jars or glass dishes
- trail mixes, nuts, fruits as well fit nicely in small jars rather than baggies

You will notice that most all processed and prepared items are packaged in some kind of plastic. By omitting these food items from your diet, you also omit so much plastic chemicals from your foods. Choose whole food items and use something other than plastic to contain or store them in.

# Chapter 11

# MICROWAVE YOUR FOOD – WHY NOT?

Microwave cooking has become very popular around the world because of its speed in cooking and heating. Most people now prefer to use the microwave over the conventional stove top and oven even though foods do not stay hot as long, foods become soggy instead of crisp, and the outcome is often less attractive and desirable. But because of convenience and habit, these reasons are usually overlooked.

Most people, however, are unaware of the harmful effects of using a microwave for cooking or heating foods. The fact is that in spite the convenience of it, microwave cooking is causing harm to your foods, and these harmful effects are passed on to YOU!

Here are some facts to consider regarding microwave cooking:

- Microwaving destroys the life-force that gives food its vitality and nourishment.
- Microwaving alters the food chemistry, which causes structural disintegration of the foods, losing 60-90 percent of the vital nutrients. Microwaving creates cancer-causing agents within foods.
- Microwave-cooked foods lower the body's ability to utilize essential vitamins and minerals, causing digestive disorders as well as the degeneration of the body's ability to protect itself against disease. [35]

In addition, microwaving your foods has been found to:

- cause brain damage
- disrupt male and female hormone production
- cause stomach and intestinal and colon growths
- cause cancerous cells to increase in the human blood
- cause immune system deficiencies through the lymph and blood
- cause loss of memory, concentration, emotional instability

"Microwaves are a form of electromagnetic energy, like light waves or radio waves, and occupy a part of the electromagnetic spectrum of power, or energy. Microwaves are very short waves of electromagnetic energy that travel at the speed of light (186,282 miles per second).

"Radiation, as defined by physics terminology, is 'the electromagnetic waves emitted by the atoms and molecules of a radioactive substance as a result of nuclear decay.' Radiation causes ionization, which is what occurs when a neutral atom gains or loses electrons. In simpler terms, a microwave oven decays and changes the molecular structure of the food by the process of radiation. Had the manufacturers accurately called them 'radiation ovens', it's doubtful they would have ever sold one, but that's exactly what a microwave oven is." [36]

Information from the manufacturers and distributors of microwave ovens will warn you of the hazards around the field of a microwave due to leaks in the door seals. However, they don't warn you about the hazards of the damaged foods from the ovens themselves, and the damage that will come from eating these foods – the fact that the body cannot recognize the nutrients that nature gives them.

Bottom line, microwave heat is not real heat! It is ruining your food even just for a short reheating time, and it can be creating diminishing health effects in you! Isn't it time to get rid of your microwave…or use it as a storage cabinet instead of for cooking?

Here are some quick and simple methods of preparing your foods without a microwave:

1) <u>Cooking or heating on a stove top:</u> Use a conventional oven stove top for cooking sauces and reheating foods. It only takes two minutes to reheat food. You just get out a saucepan, place 2-4 tablespoons of water in it, turn on the burner, add your food, and place the lid on, and it's warm in about a minute.

   *Sauces and gravies also do best on a stove top and the outcome of the food is always so much better.

2) <u>Baking or heating in a counter-top convection oven:</u> This oven beats all when it comes to defrosting or heating up foods because 1) there is no warm-up time as heat is instant, and 2) blowing combined with heat speeds up the cooking time greatly.

   *Warm up leftovers in glass or stainless steel.

   *Baking foods such as potatoes (30-35 min.), sweet potatoes (20-40 min. depending on size), baked squashes or eggplant (15-20 min.), baked fish or chicken tenders (10-15 min.), baked salmon or other fish (10-15 min.).

   *French fries or sweet potato fries (using one-quarter of the fat by just tossing cut sticks in a large bowl with a little oil and seasonings) takes 10-15 min. baking time).

3) <u>Cooking and baking in a convection oven:</u> Most new ovens have the convection cooking option which makes cooking time much faster. However, there is still the preheating time to allow for.

   *Baking potatoes (45-50 min.)

   *Cooking main dishes (10-15 min. less time than usual)

   *Baking breads of any kind (5-10 min. less time than usual)

   *Cooking meats, chicken breasts or tenders, fish fillets (10-15 min. less time than usual)

4) <u>Broiling:</u> We seem to have forgotten how fast and easy broiling is. Just turn on your oven to "broil" during your preparations, and it's ready when you are.

   *Warming tortillas for wraps or tacos (1-2 min.)

*Cooking vegetable fillets: zucchini, eggplant, potatoes (2-4 min. instead of pan-frying in a skillet)

5) <u>Steaming in a steam pot:</u> A super quick way to cook foods is through steaming, and this preserves more of your nutrients. Just place 1 inch of water in your steaming pot and turn it on while you are preparing your foods, so it is ready when you are.

6) <u>Thawing:</u> The best ways are not using any heat at all

*Breads/tortillas (remove them and separate 15-30 min. before use)

*Meats (place in a sink of warm water for 15-30 min.)

*Fruits for eating (place in a bowl in a sink full of warm water for 5-10 min.

# Chapter 12

# THE BODY'S SEVEN CHANNELS OF ELIMINATION

Your body has seven systems that work to eliminate waste and toxic substances. A wholesome diet, plenty of pure water, and exercise are all important in helping these systems work efficiently so you can enjoy great health. Understanding these seven channels of elimination help you recognize what is going on in your body when your system is challenged and how to proceed to support and correct it.

Detoxification and cleansing internally on a regular basis is essential to your overall health. As you cleanse, it is vitally important that you keep these channels open, free flowing and functioning optimally.

The body has primary and secondary channels of elimination:

## Primary channels

- Colon, intestinal tract
- Kidneys, urinary system
- Liver plays a huge role in each of these systems

## Secondary channels

- Skin
- Lungs, respiratory system
- Blood, circulatory system
- Lymphatic system

COLON: Your colon is vital for effective health as it transports solid waste out of the body. Plenty of water, fiber, and water-rich produce contribute to improving colon health and its functioning optimally.

KIDNEYS: Your kidneys are responsible for removing the liquid waste from your body. Again proper hydration with pure water is important.

LIVER: Your liver is king! It is one of the largest and most important organs in your body providing many functions. It metabolizes food, filters toxins, converts ingredients into substances needed for all body parts, it stores vitamins, fats, sugars, and other nutrients, builds chemicals that your body needs, breaks down harmful substances, removes waste from your blood, and makes sure your body has the constituents it needs to be healthy.

SKIN: Your skin is the largest organ in the body and largest channel of elimination. With regular exercise and sweating, pure water, and good foods, you assist your body in drawing out many toxins and impurities.

LUNGS: The best way you can take care of your lungs is by exercising in clean open air (not traffic pollution, smoking environment, etc.) and avoiding environmental toxicity. Deep breathing exercises two to three times daily for a few minutes are also helpful.

BLOOD: Your blood transfers and transports substances throughout your body, both nutrients needed to body parts and removing toxic waste.

LYMPHATIC SYSTEM: The lymphatic system is the body's filtration system, filtering out bacteria and foreign particles. This system has no pump. To stimulate proper flow requires: exercise, water, massage, and/or essential oils.

Now here is the huge Secret... As you look at your primary and secondary pathways of elimination, ask yourself what might be happening if you are experiencing "seasonal allergies"?

Your respiratory system is your secondary pathway of elimination, so if your respiratory system is being challenged, this means your digestive system is overloaded and can't handle the stress. Thus, the secondary pathway is taking on the challenge.

You can address the respiratory system all you want (the Western mentality), however, until you address the primary pathways – your digestive system – you will continue to experience the discomfort from these allergies. This is why cleansing is so beneficial.

Let's really understand this again…once your primary pathways (default systems) are being challenged and stressed, by design, your body has other pathways that carry the burden – your skin and your lungs (also your blood and lymph). With this understanding, you know that if you are having skin and lung issues (secondary pathways of elimination) your digestive system (primary pathways of elimination: colon, kidneys, liver) are working overtime with too much toxicity to handle the load. Most people think of skin issues as a topical issue – when in reality, cleansing the liver, colon, and kidneys are the important area of focus.

I speak from experience. With my initial lifestyle change – whole foods, several cleanses, balanced supplements, herbal medicines – I realized two years later that I no longer had the seasonal allergies. I was so glad to say goodbye to allergies forever! And over thirty years later, I have not experienced allergies except for a couple of short experiences when breathing in dust or smoke. CLEANSING is vital – not just one time, but on a continual basis. Follow the 90-Day Cleanse – make sure you are intent on being precise – you will forever love the benefits!

In addition, there are so many misconceptions when it comes to energy in today's world. So many people struggle with fibromyalgia, chronic pain, depression, lack of energy, and they buy into the lies that energy drinks, energy bars, and medications will somehow bring their body from disorder to order, producing the health and energy they are seeking.

True energy and wellness come from having a CLEAN SYSTEM. Just like a car – you've learned that providing good care for your car, you must give it the proper fuel, have regular filter and oil changes, and tune ups. Doing this will not only minimize sluggishness and help it run more efficiently; it will also extend the life of your car. Why not understand this concept for your own body?

Although you can't "drain the oil and replace it with new" as you do on your car, you can provide your body with proper fuel and cleanse your filtration systems on a continual basis. A concept that's good for your car is even more important for your body.

However, the biggest difference is that the body toxicity goes cellular... brain fog is a toxicity issue, obesity is a toxicity issue, heart disease is a toxicity issue, joint pain is a toxicity issue, and so on. Your body likes and requires healthy happy cells for order to take place. Polluted cells produce disorder!

Going on a simple cleanse won't produce overnight results – another misconception. If you are determined to cleanse the impurities and toxicity from your body, you've got to go all the way to the cellular level and that means you initially need to do several different cleanses, apply certain principles, and be in it for the long haul for the long-term benefits. Remember, true principles will only benefit you as long as you apply them. Real energy is for you as you understand the importance of cleansing!

# Chapter 13

# WATER,
# THE PURE AND
# PERFECT CLEANSER

My friend Pauline shares her story: "In October 2013, I weighed 165 pounds (5'2"), and was stuck at that weight for more than a year, no matter what I ate or how much I exercised. (I was monitoring weight and exercise with the 'MyFitnessPal' phone app). In mid-November, I began using four drops of a metabolic essential oil blend once a day in a glass of water, and it was like my metabolism was jump started. I began losing about a pound a week for the first several months with no other changes to diet or exercise.

"The following February, I stopped all herbal supplements I had been taking for many years and added a balanced set of nutritional supplements to my daily health regimen. I continued to lose weight being consistent with my metabolic blend drops and a lot of water, but more important, I felt better and had more energy. By the end of February, I had lost about fifteen pounds, and people had started to notice and ask me how I lost the weight.

"In April, I took Erleen's Certified Holistic Wellness Coaching Class and made the decision to eat 90 percent unprocessed foods / 50 percent raw foods for the month of June. I decided to continue in July (80 percent unprocessed foods / 40 percent raw). In August, I began weekly Saturday training sessions where lots of snack foods were available; although they did have some fruit and nuts available, I succumbed to the temptation of processed cheese and crackers for three weeks in a row. That was an eye-opening experience. By the following week, I was coughing every morning with chest congestion; at that time, I made the decision to eliminate processed dairy products and resumed the unprocessed foods diet, which I continue to follow. Since then, I have continued to lose weight WITHOUT TRYING at a faster pace (five to eight pounds per month) and as of today, November 3, 2014, I weigh 125 pounds – forty pounds lighter than I was a year ago."

Foods are your Builders; Water is your Cleanser – inside and out! Every day you need to build and cleanse your body, and cleansing requires water. Not milk, not juice, soft drinks, sport drinks, coffee, or other drinks. Again, these are all acids and basically pollutants! Your body needs water!

All cells, including those on the skin, are made up of approximately 70 percent water. Water surrounds and cushions our cells in the form of interstitial fluid. This fluid protects cells, as well as transports waste from normal metabolic processes. This waste is excreted in many ways, including through the skin. Adequate water consumption is paramount for optimal cell and body function. As the body's largest organ, this holds true for skin as well. Water hydrates the skin's cells and carries nutrients throughout your body to feed various organs. As the skin is the largest organ, and one with many functions, it requires a large amount of fluid on a daily basis. Water works to flush your skin of impurities, regulate body temperature, and maintain a fresh, supple appearance. Water is the perfect calorie-free, sugar-free, cleansing agent you have.

If you are looking to release a few pounds, water will be one of your most valuable tools. And if you want to cleanse your body all the way to a cellular level, again pure clean water is vital – and lots of it!

## WHY WATER IS SO IMPORTANT

Some of the best information about water I've found comes from *Water: for Health, for Healing, for Life* and *Your Body's Many Cries for Water* by F. Batmanghelidj, MD. Here are some of the important things he brings out.

He recommends drinking a full glass of water before each meal, and if you do, "The volume of food intake will decrease drastically, the type of craving for food will also change. With sufficient water intake, we tend to crave proteins more than fattening carbohydrates. If you think you are different and your body does not need this amount of water [8-10 glasses per day], you are making a major mistake". [37]

"Every function of the body is monitored and pegged to the efficient flow of water." Water transports nutrients, lubricates, hydrates…the lack of it can be life threatening as he brings out:

"The primary cause of Alzheimer's disease is chronic dehydration of the body."

"Arthritis pain is another of the regional thirst signals of the body."

"Basically, migraine seems to be an indicator of critical body temperature regulation at times of 'heat stress'. Dehydration plays a major role in the precipitation of migraine headaches."

"With dehydration, the level of energy generation in the brain is decreased…We recognize this inadequacy of function and call it depression. This 'depressive state' caused by dehydration can lead to chronic fatigue syndrome."

"Dehydration causes stress, and stress will cause further dehydration."

"…so many millions of children suffer unnecessarily to the point of a few thousand of them dying of asthma. What these children need to realize is the fact that, for them, breathing has become difficult because they are so thirsty." [38]

The most simple and inexpensive, yet most vital parts of wellness come from just drinking good pure water…not any other drinks – just water! Experience the benefits for yourself.

## WHAT TYPE OF WATER IS BEST

There is much information available out there about which kind of water is best to drink, but here are my conclusions based on what I've experienced personally and studied:

- Tap water is not our best source of water due to contaminants, chlorine, fluoride, and other bacteria – just don't drink tap water unless it comes from a good natural spring.
- Reverse Osmosis home systems most often produce more contaminated water simply because people don't change the filters

often enough. A Reverse Osmosis filter builds up with contaminants and bacteria, and if not changed regularly, the bacteria growth can produce more dangerous levels of toxicity than the tap water to begin with.

- Reverse Osmosis commercial systems normally change their filters on a weekly basis IF they are selling hundreds of gallons consistently. Thus, you will usually find much purer water there than you will in a home system. Ask your local water store to find out how often their filters are being changed.

- Alkaline water systems may remove acidity, but they don't necessarily remove impurities. So while you may think you are getting good tasting alkaline water, you may be fooling yourself with many of the impurities still present.

- Distilled water does remove all the minerals, contaminants, and bacteria. And though some research may claim distilled water to be acidic, in truth, once ingested it has a neutral pH balance.

My recommendation is getting good water – for drinking and cooking – from either a commercial reverse osmosis system or a distilled water system. Then with either, use a good mineral salt for ALL your salt intake: Celtic, Himalayan, Real Salt, etc. and omit regular table salt from your diet (high in chlorine and other contaminants too). This way you will increase your cleansing abilities and get good mineral composition too.

## YOUR DAILY WATER INTAKE

Though covered previously, we need to reinforce this concept here again. Your body requires a minimum of approximately one-half of your body's weight in ounces daily…that's minimum, but NOT enough for cleansing. So if you weigh 150 lbs., you need to drink a minimum of 75oz. of water for daily maintenance. However, as previously stated, for cleansing and shedding a few pounds, you will need to double that amount and drink your body's weight in ounces of water daily.

Good news though. As you shed the pounds, you will be drinking less water, so drink up all you can! The other great piece of good news is that you will have more energy, think more clearly, and feel so much better. Visiting the toilet a little more often will be on the agenda. Just plan on it and be grateful that you are eliminating all those unwanted toxins that your body doesn't need every time you pee! Realistically, you can be eliminating many pounds of pure toxicity.

Now would you like to know how to learn to love drinking water AND accelerate the cleansing process – even maybe about ten times? Add lemon essential oil to your water. But wait, be careful. All essential oils are not created equally. Most every lemon essential oil on the market smells like furniture polish and is NOT safe for internal use and may only create additional toxicity. Make sure you choose only pure therapeutic-grade essential oils that are guaranteed safe for internal use. A pure lemon essential oil will make you will think you are smelling the rind of an organic lemon.

Lemon essential oil is a power house for cleansing the body as you remember in reading Jenni's story. Though one of the least expensive of oils, it can have such a powerful effect in cleansing your internal self. Because essential oils are lipophilic in composition, they can easily penetrate the cellular wall. Lemon essential oil can assist the body in exporting contaminants and petrochemicals from the cells. Grapefruit essential oil - which is really tasty as well – is also a powerhouse for cleansing as well as shrinking your fat cells. In reality, other citrus essential oils can also provide some cleansing benefits (though maybe not as much) so on occasion consider also using lime, orange, bergamot, or a blend of these.

At the beginning of each day, fill your glass water containers according to what you want and need to consume on a daily basis. This helps you keep track of how much you are actually drinking. Juice bottles and vinegar bottles make great water bottles. DO NOT add essential oils to plastic water bottles or cups – only use glass. Stainless steel isn't even recommended.

Next add drops of lemon or grapefruit essential oil to your containers (or others on occasion), consuming according to your own taste: ten to twenty drops daily. You will learn to LOVE water and what it will do for you, so drink up and enjoy the benefits.

# Chapter 14

# 90-DAY CLEANSE
# WITH A 30-DAY OUTLINE

If you remember my story and where I found success in my change of health, one key principle was that after my initial mindset change, I decided that I was in it for the long haul. I wanted permanent success – I was tired of not feeling well – so I committed to making permanent changes in my habits, my lifestyle, and my future. Because of this, within a few short months, the difference in how I felt was life-changing for me. I knew that whole foods, cleansing and all of the other principles (that you are yet to learn) was where real health is found. Had I only "tried" this thing for a couple of weeks or even a month, I don't think I would have ever found the success that I did.

So consider for yourself:

- a 90-day cleanse for thorough cellular cleansing benefits
- making permanent changes in your lifestyle and habits
- going for the long haul and truly experiencing the lifestyle of healthy happy people
- specifically following the Cleansing Diet in Chapter 29

You have one more thing to consider as you contemplate this 90-Day Cleansing program. Over thirty years ago when I did my initial cleanse and restore program, I was at the mercy of a naturopathic physician who had a variety of resources that he felt were beneficial – and they were. They didn't come from a specific line of products, just a la carte from different sources and who knows where. The cost of those supplements for cleansing and building my body ranged from $250 - $300 monthly. Again, this was MORE than my house payment at that time! Could I really afford this on a young marrieds' budget with only my spouse bringing in the cash flow? The real question at that point was, could I afford NOT to do this? This was my body and my future. I trusted in his professional advice, and it paid off – I will forever be grateful for his mentorship and guidance!

Today people spend ALL KINDS OF MONEY for health emergencies, yet they are reluctant to spend money to avoid the emergencies to begin with. Do yourself a favor and do this cleanse, find the money somewhere – just as you would if it was an emergency. If you follow through with exactness, you will reap the benefits!

## Foundational Cleansing Supplements and Techniques

**Organ Cleansing**: Daily support for all 90 days

A good organ cleanse that targets both the primary and secondary pathways of elimination is important. The colon, kidneys, liver, skin and lungs need daily cleansing support to work optimally. Essential oils that support cleansing the organs include geranium, juniper berry, cilantro, rosemary, and citrus oils. They can be taken internally if they are guaranteed safe for internal use, which will provide great internal benefits, or they can be applied topically over the liver, kidneys, abdomen or bottoms of feet. These are powerful essential oils, yet mild enough to consume almost daily for ongoing cleansing as needed.

**Herbal Organ Cleansing**: Daily support for all 90 days

An herbal cleansing blend which includes psyllium, dandelion, red clover, and other herbs will complement the cleansing process for your five organs. These especially support your primary pathways of elimination: colon, liver and kidney, which are so foundational in your overall health.

**Digestive Enzyme Complex**: Support for all 90 days

This is usually one of the most important pieces in a cleanse. Most mature adults do not get enough enzymes to begin with, so they don't digest well. Here's how a digestive enzyme can greatly help you in a cleanse:

2 capsules upon arising
2-3 capsules with breakfast
2 capsules mid to late morning
2-3 capsules with lunch
2 capsules mid to late afternoon
2-3 capsules with dinner

That's 12-15 capsules per day. This action will break down the matter in the intestines and will provide excellent cleansing support. After the first 30 days, you can cut your doses in half if you feel the need. However, if you are quite toxic and need to lose weight, it will pay to stick with this regime for 90 days and then go to the recommended doses. Two first thing in the morning is still helpful in moving the bowels.

**Balanced Micronutrient Supplements**: Daily Support for all 90 days

For cleansing and natural weight release, unless you are getting the proper amount of balanced, whole-food nutrition in a cellular delivery system, you won't get the same benefits. For overall health and releasing pounds, balanced supplements are a must, not an option. Be choosy and go for the best.

**Gallstone/Liver Cleanse**: Great for Day 1-2, repeat on Day 31 and Day 61. This is a great cleanse to jump start cleansing your organs.

1) For breakfast, eat a piece of fresh fruit, or fruit and vegetable smoothie. Drink loads of water throughout the day, minimum 3 quarts, preferably more.
2) Every two hours on the hour after breakfast, drink 1/2 organic lemon squeezed into 8 ounces distilled water alternately with 8 oz. unfiltered apple juice (no other foods throughout the day)
3) At 6 p.m., take 5-6 herbal psyllium-based organ cleanse capsules, which will create a laxative effect. You need to promote increased bowel cleansing. Drink lots of water.
4) At 8:00 pm, drink 1 cup lukewarm water with 1 Tablespoon Epsom salt in it.
5) At bedtime, combine 1/2 cup olive oil and 1/2 cup lemon juice or grapefruit juice. Don't take this until crawling into bed.

6) Lie down on your right side and lie still for at least two hours.

7) Upon arising, drink 1 cup lukewarm water with 1 Tablespoon Epsom salt in it to flush your digestive tract. You should be dispelling many strange-looking items in the toilet like you've never seen before.

8) To increase the effects, enemas or colonics on day 2 are highly recommended.

9) Continue to drink water throughout the day, but you can resume with meals that include many fresh fruits and vegetables.

## Lemon Liver Detox: Continue after Gallstone/Liver Cleanse

This detox in addition provides major cleansing of the liver and can be taken daily up to 14 days. Combine the juice from 1 organic lemon, 10 drops each lemon and peppermint essential oils (meant for internal use only), in 8 ounces of purified water. Drink all at once upon rising, and include lots of water throughout your day.

## GI Cleanse: Start on Day 11 through Day 20

Because of unhealthy bacteria and residue that builds in the gut especially due to processed foods, milk products, breads, etc., this cleanse can be really beneficial. Note that the foods that rot in your intestines are the same foods that you crave, so removing the bacteria will usually remove your cravings. Combined essential oils such as oregano, melaleuca, lemon, lemongrass, peppermint, and thyme are very effective in removing gut bacteria. Since oregano and these other essential oils are powerful, 10 days is the maximum amount of time for this cleanse. To accelerate the process, do this along with the Candida Cleanse (below). After 10 days, stop taking this combination of oils and start taking a good probiotic for a minimum of 10 days as well to replenish the gut with good sources of healthy flora and provide ongoing digestive support.

## Candida Cleanse: Also start on Day 11 through Day 20

Excess Candida microorganisms can be produced in the gut due to a diet rich in sugar, processed foods, milk products, white breads, coffee, and tea. Sugar especially depresses your immune system, which more readily allows the Candida yeast to proliferate. Antibiotics can also create excess Candida as it kills the friendly bacteria along with the harmful.

A Candida cleanse can be highly beneficial if followed in this manner:

1) Commit to a 10 day period of following these instructions faithfully – don't cheat!
2) Eliminate ALL fruits, honey or other sweeteners, grains, potatoes, sweet potatoes, carrots, peanuts and other nuts (except almonds), most beans, all milk products, vinegar, coffee, black tea, alcohol and tobacco of any kind.
3) You can eat an abundance of vegetables and greens, raw almond butter, raw almonds (or soaked), eggs, lean chicken or fish, coconut oil and other fats, liquid stevia (only sweetener), herbal teas, avocados…think lots of salads with protein, green smoothie with stevia, lettuce wraps, soups, grilled meats… and a 101 ways to eat vegetables :). Snack time: celery and almond butter or hummus (on occasion).
4) Include a good digestive enzyme as suggested.
5) Follow the GI Cleanse.
6) Make sure you are drinking lots of water and no other drinks, and you are including exercise in your daily routine.
7) After the 10-day period, stop taking the essential oils combination with peppermint, oregano, etc. and follow up with taking a good probiotic.

**Probiotic**: Day 21-30 following GI Cleanse, can continue except when doing the GI

Now that you have cleansed the intestines of candida and unhealthy bacteria, it's important to replenish it with an abundance of friendly flora. Choose a probiotic that is live and will preferably be in a delivery system that will make it all the way to the intestines. Many probiotics are highly concentrated due to compensate of losing 80-90 percent of it in the stomach. Keep in mind that replenishing your gut with good intestinal flora should be an ongoing focus for good digestion.

**Lemon and Metabolic Essential Oil Blends**: Daily following Lemon

Liver Detox

Add essential oils to your water to increase cleansing action such as lemon or a metabolic blend. Again, the secret to having optimal energy is having a clean system, and lemon will be so helpful on a cellular level. A metabolic blend including lemon, grapefruit, ginger, peppermint, and cinnamon will increase your digestion and overall metabolism, which will also increase your energy naturally. Keep in mind that you can also apply essential oils topically too. Grapefruit essential oil is excellent for reducing cellulite with topical applications.

After the 30-day period, repeat twice. If you do the full 90-day cleanse, your energy will greatly increase, your mental health will improve, seasonal allergies and other ailments will most likely disappear. You will feel like a totally different person! It's so worth it!!

# Chapter 15

# HYDROTHERAPY

A few years ago, a neighbor friend of ours came down with hepatitis and reached out for help. My friend and I put our heads together...she came up with a nutrition protocol, and I sought out a remedy for a detox. My research led me to an Epsom Salt bath detox, which included Epsom Salt and three essential oils: peppermint, eucalyptus, and melaleuca. I carefully combined them together in a large jar and dropped them by with instructions for him: Soak twice daily for approximately fifteen minutes in very warm bath water with ½ cup or more of the bath salts. The results were amazing! He reported that each time after soaking, the bath water was the color of a yellow crayon! He contributed to his quick recovery to this detox protocol!

In addition to drinking plenty of pure water and doing some intense internal cleansing, here are some great suggestions to enhance the cleansing process. As you read along, see how these might benefit you and others in different situations.

1. Herbal infusions: As the proper name for herbal teas (tea is a plant, not a preparation), herbal infusions are alkalizing, highly beneficial for cleansing and hydrating the body, calming, invigorating, improving digestion, and providing nutrient support and benefits: peppermint, chamomile, elder flowers and more are great. With any herbal infusion (tea) preparation, I like to add 1-2 drops cinnamon essential oil – it's so yummy and excellent for digestion and balancing your blood sugar.

2. Hot showers: Oftentimes, clogged pores and ducts can open up in a comfortably hot shower, especially in the case of clogged sinuses or mastitis. Wintergreen essential oil also helps mastitis and can help

relieve the inflammation, while peppermint or eucalyptus essential oils help support the sinuses.

3. Baths/Jacuzzi: Epsom salts baths are excellent for sore muscles, inflammation, the coming on of a virus, stress reduction, fever reduction, after-delivery sitz baths, and more. Here is a basic recipe for <u>Cleansing Bath Salts</u> (the one used for my hepatitis friend above): 2 C. Epsom salt, 10-12 drops of each eucalyptus, peppermint, and melaleuca essential oils. Add to glass jar and shake well to mix thoroughly; add ⅓-½ cup to each bath. Other essential oils can be used instead for specific desired results. For aches, pains, and stimulation, a Jacuzzi is also helpful.

4. Foot Baths: A hot foot bath is considered the most basic and most commonly used of all hydrotherapy techniques and is very simple and convenient. It also has profound physiological effects that have been demonstrated through research, knowing that the feet have the largest pores on the body. Make sure to use pure water, and add the above <u>Cleansing Bath Salts</u> or other for optimal benefits.

5. Saunas / Steam Inhalation: Sweating is the body's safe and natural way to heal. Scientists and doctors are finally acknowledging what our ancestors instinctively knew, that regular sweating restores good health through the elimination of toxins. Sweating has proven its effectiveness in flushing out toxins and disease and maintaining optimal physical as well as mental health.

6. Enemas: An enema is a health procedure wherein you gently force water or another liquid solution into your bowels through your anus to loosen fecal matter other impacted material, and cleanse out unwanted bacteria. The health benefits of an enema vary and generally depend on the solution used. Many recipes exist for various health conditions that may include apple cider vinegar or lemon juice (2 Tbs. per quart pure water), herbal infusions (chamomile, burdock root, etc.), or essential oils (see below for details).

7. Hot/cold wet compresses: A hot compress is recommended for chronic conditions such as tight muscles, menstrual cramps, and arthritic pain. Apply a cold compress after a recent, soft-tissue injury

such as a sprain, pulled ligament or an overextended muscle by wrapping the injured body part in a cold compress every two hours for at least 20 minutes. Hot or cold compresses should never be directly next to the skin. Applying 1-2 drops of essential oil on the area prior to adding the compress greatly accelerates the healing and recovery process.

8. Neti Pot to address sinus infection and symptoms:

- 2 drops Lavender essential oil
- 2 drops Melaleuca essential oil
- 2 drops Rosemary essential oil

Apply topically with a cotton swab inside the nostrils or mix the above with a cup of warm water and, using a Neti pot (nasal irrigation device available at most drug stores) irrigate the nasal passages.

To address sinus infection and symptoms (heavy duty):

- 3 drops Eucalyptus essential oil
- 2 drops Rosemary essential oil
- 2 drops Frankincense essential oil
- 1 teaspoons sea salt

Mix the above with 2 cups of warm water and, using a Neti pot (nasal irrigation device available at most drug stores) irrigate 2 times per day (or more).

## Enemas or Colonics

Several years back, my neighbor contacted me with concern about her 18-month-old son. He had been having diarrhea for about four weeks now, and she did not know what to do. The week prior, he had been in the hospital for several days, and now that he was back home a few days, he still had the diarrhea. She wanted to know if I had any suggestions. My first suggestion was an enema, and she freaked out! His stool was runny – that seemed to just add to the problem in her mind. I explained to her that there were obviously some unhealthy bacteria in his colon that was being circulated, and it needed to be cleansed from his system.

I offered to help her and do the enema. With just one dose of water solution in his colon – he was much too wiggly to tie down to do any more – followed by dissolving one capsule of acidophilus in one tablespoon of water and inserting that back into the rectum after he expelled the water solution, the diarrhea was gone and over! That was all it took!

I had learned with my own son, who had asthma as a young child. Giving him an enema was like pulling the plug. So much mucous came out in the toilet, and afterward, he could breathe.

One of my other children when young had an unending cough that carried on for two months. My chiropractor told me that she obviously had bacteria in her colon that was being reabsorbed back into her system, and that an enema would help. I was amazing how fast the cough went away after an enema. Not the most fun thing to do, but for her sake, I wished I had administered it over a month earlier.

Enemas can be effective for cleansing the body for an infection, worms (parasites), fever, mucous and colds, dehydration, diarrhea, constipation, etc., though it is not recommended on a frequent basis except for a healing crisis.

The colon is the waste basket of the system, where all your toxic waste settles and must be discarded. Sometimes it becomes clogged and does not clean out properly, and oftentimes is the very reason for an illness. Unwanted bacteria and waste accumulate on the walls of the intestines, and even begin to form pockets of built-up layers of this waste, especially with a diet of highly processed foods, which are depleted of the necessary roughage to cleanse it out. If this toxic matter gets compacted in the colon, as is often the case, toxicity is continually absorbed into the blood system reintroducing unhealthy and unwanted impurities. Therefore again, your diet is a contributing factor to your health and your colon.

Enemas are not to be afraid of and can be administered in a relaxed manner, whether for yourself or for someone else. There are several types of enema bulbs or bags – bulbs for babies and children, and bags for adults. For babies and children, make sure to get one with a very small tip as not to add discomfort. Never use a petroleum product for lubrication, but instead use coconut oil. Before using, always thoroughly sterilize enema bag, tip, hose, and containers used with alcohol, then hot soapy water, then sterilize again when completely done. There are several solutions that can be used for enemas (see below). Lying on the floor on your right side, with a towel underneath and a pillow under head for support, if desired, insert lubricated tip into rectum and allow solution from enema bag or bulb to fill colon only until slightly uncomfortable. Lightly massage upward on left side of belly then across at waistline until water is unable to hold further (not more than a minute or two). Expel in toilet and repeat process. Flushing out the colon is a time-consuming process, which is most beneficial when done five to eight times in one session (colonics take much less time and provide more thorough flushings). Oftentimes, children only have the patience for three to four flushings, but every bit helps.

## Enema Solutions

For most adults, 2 quarts water prepared is the ideal. For children will need only 1-4 cups depending on age. For 1 quart of room temperature, purified water you can add:

- 1-2 tablespoons apple cider vinegar or fresh squeezed lemon juice, or
- 2-3 drops lemon or cypress essential oils work great

Repeat as needed.

# OIL PULLING

Oil pulling is a safe and simple way to bring health to your mouth and to your body by pulling harmful toxins and bacteria out of your body. Dentists will tell you that disease begins in the mouth, and your mouth is a blueprint of the health of your body, which is why this is a great technique.

Oil pulling has been a practice in Ayurvedic medicine for many years and has shown remarkable results with illnesses such as headaches, bronchitis, diseased teeth, leukemia, arthritis, paralysis, eczema, heart disease, kidney disease, woman's hormonal dysfunctions, stroke, diabetes, and more.

According to Dr. Mercola, "Candida and Streptococcus are common residents in your mouth, and these germs and their toxic waste products can contribute to plaque accumulation and tooth decay. Oil pulling may help lessen the overall toxic burden on your immune system by preventing the spread of these organisms from your mouth to the rest of your body, by way of your bloodstream." [39]

People are finding more and more benefits from oil pulling for addressing certain diseases, possibly extending your life, and even whitening your teeth in the process. It is a process that is completely harmless and so inexpensive for the benefits it provides.

Here is the basic procedure:

1) Do this first thing in the morning after arising and brushing your teeth
2) Take 2-3 teaspoons of coconut oil (other oils may work but coconut oils is found to be a superior choice) with a few added drops of essential oil (see chart that follows) and put it into your mouth.
3) Swish, pull, and push oil between your teeth (you can do this while showering, getting dressed, doing your facial skin care routine, etc.) and do not swallow!
4) Spit out the oil – DO NOT SWALLOW any of it! Now that you have pulled all the toxins from your mouth, you want to discard all of it. In addition, if you are using regular coconut oil, discard it in the garbage can liner, not the toilet or sink or you may clog your plumbing.
5) Take extra time to brush your teach and scrape your tongue to remove any trace of toxicity as possible.

You can add any essential oil but specific ones can provide specific benefits such as:

- Birch / Wintergreen – restoring enamel and dentin on teeth
- Clove – mouth and gum health, analgesic, anti-biotic, and antiseptic
- Frankincense – analgesic, cold, flu, mouth trauma, antiseptic, anti-inflammatory
- Geranium – mouth and gum health, throat, laryngitis, analgesic, antiseptic
- Grapefruit – cleansing, detoxifying, anti-septic, antibacterial
- Lemon – cleansing, detoxifying, cold, sore throat, anti-septic
- Lemongrass – herpes, halitosis

- Melaleuca – cold, flu, immune support, braces irritation, gum and mouth sores, congestion, herpes, anti-inflammatory, anti-bacterial, antiseptic
- Myrrh – mouth, teeth and gum, cold, flu, tonsillitis, anti-inflammatory, anti-bacterial, antiseptic
- Oregano – flu, virus, sore throat, swollen glands, cold sores, herpes, anti-inflammatory, anti-bacterial, antibiotic, anti-viral

Give it a try as you will find some kind of benefits although probably not noticeable after only done once or twice.

## GOALS AND SUGGESTIONS

If you want to be free of many bodily dysfunctions, then you have to STOP polluting your body and start nourishing and cleansing it consistently. Can you stop today and make that shift? YES! I did it – you can do it! Decide that wellness and energy is what you want, and as I said earlier – make it a permanent lifestyle change. If you want to live like healthy happy people, you've got to DO what healthy happy people do. They nourish and cleanse on a daily basis.

1. Start by adding pure, therapeutic lemon, grapefruit or other essential oil to the water that you are carefully measuring out in ounces according to your body weight in glass bottles. Remember no plastic water bottles, just glass. Drink this throughout the day so you can get the amount of water you need.

2. Start the 90-day Cleanse. If you would like help and have a mentor to guide you through this program, please visit: www.livingahealthylifestyle.com.

# BUILD

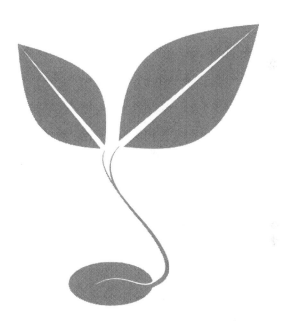

# Chapter 16

# BALANCED NUTRITION

When I had my own life-changing experience as a young mother, with all the changes that I made in my lifestyle choices, I believe that a balanced source of nutrients was one of the most powerful aspects of pulling me out of that deep dark pit. I needed a change of diet, I had to cleanse the toxicity from my body, and I needed nature's medicines for some of the conditions I was experiencing, but what I believe ultimately gave my body the ability to become whole and well again was concentrated, balanced nutrition through good quality supplements.

I see many others that have had similar experiences with many different challenges. The bottom line is that balanced sources of our *micro*nutrients have been a key support for so many individuals.

Read what Carey shares: "Fifteen years ago, when I was seven months pregnant with my third child, I woke up one morning, got out of bed, and could not stand upright. I was bent over at the hips and in excruciating pain. This was my first experience with my back going out. I went to the doctor, who sent me to the physical therapist, and over the next several days with a routine of rest, ice, and stretching exercises, I was upright once again. "Whew," I thought. "Glad that's over!" Little did I know that this was only the beginning of a chronic issue. From that point forward, every several months, my lower back would tighten up, and my spine would drop diagonally, offsetting my shoulders from my hips by a good six inches.

"I became a faithful chiropractic patient, receiving adjustments every two weeks, but like clockwork, my back would go out every three months or so. In frustration, I lamented to my chiropractor, "WHY does this happen? I am doing my exercises and seeing you faithfully! Shouldn't this be resolved by now?!?" He explained that sometimes injuries from our childhood that go unaddressed until they manifest in our adulthood progress to the point that maintenance is the only option. While this was frustrating to me, I recognized the truth of what he was saying. I was in my mid-twenties before I began regular care for my spine, and my active lifestyle had certainly not been kind to my back. The overall improvement in my health with regular chiropractic care, combined with a solid strategy when my back would go out were strong enough reasons to continue on. In fact…suffering a broken back from a bike accident eight years into my chronic ordeal, I can state with absolute certainty that I owe my mobility to my wonderful chiropractor.

"Fast forward to two years ago, I was introduced to some amazing wellness products and essential oils. As I began learning about and experiencing the power of essential oils, my vision exploded with possibility. My son's anxiety, overall immune boosting, another child's warts…all quickly were resolved by identifying the right chemistries to apply to their bodies. I was thrilled with my newfound empowerment! What mom doesn't wish she could assist her family's health? As huge as I knew the possibilities with my own natural home pharmacy to be, the idea of resolving my chronic back issues didn't even occur to me. I had truly accepted that this was just how my body was going to be for the rest of my life. About three months into my journey, it dawned on me one day that my back hadn't been out recently. It was rarely even tightening up! The couple of times that it started, applying an essential oil blend for tension caused to my lower back to immediately relax. Four months had gone by, then five, then six, and I was in absolute awe and wonder.

"Initially I thought that the couple of times I had used the oils must have been what had resolved the issue…*but* the more I learned, the more I recognized that the healing had been **facilitated** by a set of synergistic supplements. It is critical to note, that I am not claiming that a product healed my back…but rather that those *supplements simply provided my body with the tools it needed…***to heal itself.**

"All disorder in the body is rooted in inflammation. This is why everything is an 'itis'. Arthritis, Bursitis, Bronchitis, Pancreatitis…and the list goes on. Inflammation is frequently rooted in oxidation and lack of nourishment on a cellular level. When you can find a way to nourish the body on the cellular level, *and* neutralize oxidation…it truly is remarkable how the body is able to respond. These supplements have clinically demonstrated to nourish the body on the cellular level in addition to providing a significant dose of potent antioxidants, resulting in comprehensive inflammation (and consequently pain) reduction.

"My story of resolution to a significant health challenge using these particular supplements is a dime a dozen. Thousands upon thousands of others have experienced similar positive impact. What's really neat is that in addition to being freed from my chronic back issue…my hypothyroid syndrome, for which I was taking a significant dose of medications for more than seven years, has also resolved! That makes more than two years since my last back ordeal and more than one year since I have taken a prescription drug! Heal the cell, and the body gets well!"

## THE STUDIES OF BARBARA REED STITT

I love the studies by Barbara Reed Stitt. My first introduction to her was her book *Food and Behavior,* which was a real eye-opening experience for me.

As a parole officer, Barbara discovered that a huge proportion of the parolees were junk food addicts, most were heavy drinkers and had no sign of live foods in their original living quarters. They were irritable, short-fused, experiencing depression, suicidal tendencies, insomnia, violence, and aggression. Her study into nutrition concluded that, "A malnourished central nervous system will inevitably lead to serious physical and behavioral problems, problems which no amount of medication or psychiatry can touch." She continued that, "Trying to correct a person's misbehavior before he or she has an adequate diet is very much like trying to ride a bicycle without filling the tires with air, or driving a car without first putting in gasoline – it won't, it can't work." [40]

Additionally she states that, "Because the brain is so vulnerable to its molecular environment, it is the most directly affected by diet." [41]This statement specifically hit home for me because I had been teaching for many years that if you correct the physical self, the emotional self will take care of itself too. She brought out that this was just the opposite… feed the brain (emotional self), and the visible consequences of brain function – behavior – will change (the physical self). That was new, but it made sense!

Barbara pursued a different method of correction in her practice that she called orthomolecular psychiatry – concentrating on the biochemical and electrical molecular processes in the central nervous system...or in other words whole foods, diet, and supplements. [42] Her program for all parole correction specifically included:

- complete removal of all processed foods such as sugar, white flour, chemicals, alcohol, etc.
- lots of fresh fruits and vegetables
- lean meat proteins
- whole grain breads
- lots of water
- complete vitamin/mineral supplements, especially B vitamins

Over her twenty years as a probation officer, she had an 80 percent success rate with the parolees she personally worked with. Of those who stuck to her recommendations of a healthy diet and supplements, there was 100 percent success (the 80 percent) as those persons were able to go back into the world and function normally without crime. Those who did not stick to her healthy recommendations, (the 20 percent) went back to crime and then subsequently back to prison.

Wow! What becomes very evident with this study is that our junk food lifestyle is self-creating crime, or these criminal tendencies. Not only that, this continues to make me ache for children as I see their sweet mothers feeding them so poorly, then punishing them so harshly for their poor behavior that they are ignorantly but ultimately responsible for. We can and must be better educated about the importance of nutrition!

Barbara went on to conduct another study with the students at the Appleton Wisconsin's alternative high school. This new program meant the installation of a new kitchen, new cooks, fresh foods, whole-grain breads, and the removal of the soda and candy machines on campus.

The program for students and staff provided:

- Breakfast including whole-grain, flax-enriched bagels or bread, or whole-grain cereals, lots of fresh fruits, and a flax energy drink
- Lunch included a salad bar/ buffet with lots of fruits and vegetables, only whole-grain breads, lean meats, steamed vegetables, and occasionally baked chips
- Two energy drinks (which included high anti-oxidant juices and flax oil – high in omega-3 for brain functions)
- 8 glasses of water throughout the day

By making subtle changes in everyone's diet, Barbara said the students and teachers noticed a dramatic difference. One teacher reported during the first year of the program that students and staff noticed:

- an increased ability to concentrate
- to think more clearly
- fewer health complaints
- more self confidence
- fewer discipline referrals
- decreased tardiness
- reduced feeling of hunger
- less moodiness
- more practice of good nutrition outside of school

But here were the notable results from school officials:

- after the program, there were: 0 dropouts, 0 drug cases, 0 expulsions, 0 counts of violence
- behavior improved
- students had more concentration and more self-confidence
- there was increased academic learning
- more calmness, alert and focused
- there was notable improved teacher/student relationships
- and get this... it was less expensive as they were able to cut out the reform programs and problems due to violence, drugs, etc. [43]

Vitamin, minerals, and other nutrients are the tools that help your body function properly. Without them in balance, you can suffer emotionally, physically, mentally, and spiritually. Think about the difference it made in the parolees and in these students! Think of how this might make a difference in you and those around you!

# EPIGENITICS

In 2000, a groundbreaking genetic experiment by Randy Jirtle, a professor of radiation oncology at Duke University, and his postdoctoral student Robert Waterland set out to see if nutrition could change the genetic legacy of a particular group of mice. These mice were bright yellow, fat as pincushions, and susceptible to life-threatening diseases such as diabetes and cancer, yet with a change of the mother's diet before conception, their offspring were slender, darker brown and not susceptible to the cancer and diabetes. In other words, the effects of the agouti gene, which affects color and patterns, had been altered by diet.

The diet of these mother mice included methyl donors, commonly found in root vegetables: beets, onions, garlic, and in supplements for pregnant mothers. Being consumed by the mother mice, the methyl donors were passed into the developing embryos' chromosomes and onto the critical agouti gene. Methyl donors are small chemical clusters that can attach to a gene, creating a chemical switch that dimmed the typical harmful effects, thus making a dramatic impact on the gene expression of the baby. This study showed how changes can be made in the epigenome.

Our DNA is made up of over 25,000 genes that are regarded as the instruction book for the human body. Each of our genes has codes, chemical markers and switches that switch on or off the expression of particular genes. In order to improve our understanding of what drives human development and disease, epigenetic researchers have made great progress in understanding that the epigenome is like a complex software code, with molecular sequences and patterns that determine these switches. The epigenome is just as critical as DNA to the healthy development of organisms and very sensitive to cues from the environment. In reality, an increase of nutrients, exposure to toxins and chemicals, and other environmental factors can alter the software in the genes that not only affect the growing fetus, your brain and body for life, but most important, could affect the health and behavior of your great-grandchildren.

These studies and other epigenetics researchers conclude that our diet, behavior, and environment could have a far greater effect on our health and posterity much more than we realize. Realistically an extra bit of vitamin, a brief exposure to a toxin can tweak the epigenome, thereby alter our software genes that can affect us for life. Our lifestyle choices are important not only for enjoying a vibrant healthy life, but also taking the responsibility for how it can impact our future generations. [44]

Think about it. Have you ever considered your lifestyle choices and how they can affect your posterity physically, mentally, and emotionally?

Additionally, our Western mentality and upbringing have brainwashed us into thinking that everything health wise that happens to us can simply be blamed on our hereditary, instead of taking responsibility for our own choices. The truth of the matter is that you have a LOT of control over your health destiny. You can choose health or sickness, for the most part, through your choices of foods, supplements, and lifestyle habits.

## THE NEED FOR BALANCED NUTRITION

A report in the *Journal of Complimentary Medicine* in 2001 pointed out that US and UK government statistics show a decline in trace minerals of up to 76 percent in fruit and vegetables over the period 1940 to 1991. [45]

We can thank our commercial farmers, who don't quite understand that chemical fertilizers do not replace the nutrients being taken from the soil. And if those nutrients are not being replaced, no matter how hard we may work to get the needed nutrition from our fresh whole foods, the sorry truth is that it just isn't there. Growing or shopping organic is a step in the right direction, but the fact is that we need supplements to make up for the nutrient deficiencies not possible otherwise.

What you should look for in a quality daily supplement:

1. *Must be 100 percent free of synthetics*: The synthetic versions of vitamins and antioxidants are only "similar" to those found in nature, and they do not provide the same health benefits and can oftentimes offer adverse effects. Look for a supplement company that uses

only whole food extracts and naturally derived *micro*nutrients and ingredients.

2. *Balance is a necessity*: Taking supplements a la cart is usually perceived by the body as a chemical or drug. Let's take for example, taking large doses (2000mg) of ascorbic acid, Vitamin C. This is not in balance with other nutrients, may or may not be in a food form, and nutrients are not working together in a team-like fashion. Isolates are just a one-man team. Taking in nutrients in the proportions nature intended is very important. Look for a supplement that is clinically tested to be in the perfect range needed for your body (not too little, not too much) with a wide array of carefully balanced vitamins, minerals, enzymes, trace elements, antioxidants, phytonutrients, and essential fatty acids.

3. *Formulated for maximum absorption and digestibility:* It's not enough to get healthy supplement components. Your body must be able to absorb and utilize them on a cellular level, and this has a lot to do with the formulation. When essential oils are included in the formulation, it enhances the digestive and absorption abilities so your body can utilize the nutrients at the cellular level.

With these three factors in place, you can ensure better results in meeting your body's needs. Keep in mind that supplements are the tools to fill in where you are out of balance; therefore, be consistent and nourish your body on a daily basis.

My friend Julie shared her story:

"I have had trouble with my knees for quite some time. I am a heavier woman, and this doesn't help. I had a fall back in November 2012, and my knees were so bad that I went to visit a surgeon. He told me I didn't need to have surgery yet but most likely within the next year. I started to look up information on knee issues and what might benefit my situation. I started rubbing an essential oil pain blend on my knee every day. This was helping, but I still was not being able to take stairs of any kind without my knees having major pain. So I decided to try a balanced micronutrient set of supplements. Within a week of my taking these supplements, I was not feeling the pain in my knee. I didn't think anything of it until I skipped taking it for a few days, and all the aches and pains in my body came back. I realized how much the nutrition had been helping me.

"Also, I have tried multiple times to get myself to quit drinking soda. I was drinking at least 52oz of Diet Coke every day. It helped me take the edge (stress) off my day. Some of the positions I have held in the past at my jobs have been very stressful, and I was not being successful in getting off the soda. I had tried everything and was still having those cravings every day to have a soda. I had been to a class, and they recommended a body cleanse. So I decided it wouldn't hurt to just cleanse my body of everything. I started taking a GI cleanse, enzymes, and kept up with the balanced micronutrient supplements as recommended. After three days, my soda tasted very nasty. I stopped drinking them. I got completely off soda for about six months or more. Now every now and again, I will have a soda but not often, nor am I addicted to them any longer. I feel so much better overall."

I love her story, which clearly displays her body's need for balanced nutrition and cleansing the toxicity. Once those were in place, not only did her pain go away, her stress was reduced, and she was able to get control of her addiction too…with balanced supplements!

# Chapter 17

# MACRONUTRIENTS VS. MICRONUTRIENTS

Let's go back to what we learned in Chapter 1 about **The Daily Basic 10:**

1) Proteins – building blocks, important for growth and repair of tissue
2) Carbohydrates – the body's source of fuel and energy
3) Fats – supports, protects, lubricates and insulates the body, vital for brain food
4) Fiber – a must for moving our food and waste through the intestines
5) Vitamins – for normal cell function, growth, development
6) Minerals – essential for bones and all human bodily functions
7) Enzymes – providing catalytic action aiding digestion
8) Antioxidants – protection for our cells from free radical damage
9) Probiotics – providing good intestinal floral to keep digestion in check
10) Water – essential for cleansing inside and out

This list includes *macro*nutrients, *micro*nutrients, and water.

Macronutrients are the structural components of the foods that provide calories and energy. They include *carbohydrates, fats, proteins,* and *fiber.*

Micronutrients are the *vitamins, minerals and trace elements, enzymes, antioxidants* and *probiotics* that are, in essence, your essential micro tools for order and good health. They may have a minimal presence in your body, yet they have a massive impact on your health.

Water, as we have learned, is another essential component for keeping the body in proper cleansing order.

# BALANCED MICRONUTRIENT STUDY

The following are three different health challenges that many people are experiencing today. Several individuals participated in a sixty-day study to see what results might take place when consuming pure balanced supplements and one essential oil or oil blend on a daily consistent basis. Here are the reports from one of the individuals in each of the categories of study:

## Depression

Erinn from California reports: "At the beginning of the study, my anxiety and depression were most severe in the evening and lower in the morning. My energy and depression levels varied, as low as a 3 upon waking, but sometimes crashing to a 10 by late afternoon.

"My first week went like this:

Morning depression was low, wake early and easily, usually around six. This is usually when I feel okay these days. I get most done in the morning.

By noon, it was high, hard to stick to tasks. After ten o'clock, I started to get tired. Not as productive as I used to be. Hard to focus and stay motivated. Give up or get frustrated by things easily.

Evening depression got worse after three in the afternoon. Sometimes I cry. Will go to bed for a few hours and wake up when my boyfriend gets home. Will often feel discouraged and hopeless, don't like being alone.

"During the following seven weeks, I still had ups and downs, but there was a steady decrease in afternoon and evening anxiety and depression. I also noticed improved stability in my blood sugar levels and decreased cravings for sugar, alcohol, and wheat products. I have had trouble with food binges in the past, especially during PMS. Symptoms of PMS improved significantly as well.

"Under the guidance of my doctor, I was able to taper off two of my medications that were prescribed for anxiety, depression, and PTSD (Paxil and Risperdal). I have been able to stay off those medications since and have cut the dose of a third medication (clonopin) in half. The clonopin is going to be harder to kick, as it is very addictive, but I have faith I will eventually be off it as well. It will just take time to heal.

"At the start of the study I was struggling to concentrate on tasks that involved a lot of reading and writing. In week 7 I noted that I have been able to study more, still best early to mid-morning. I am finally making some progress on an online personal training course. I signed up for this class last March. By midsummer, my depression was so bad I quit working on it and requested an extension. I feel like I am back on track and have a plan to complete the course by May.

"By week 8 my energy levels were staying fairly stable throughout the entire day, between 2 and 4. Energy has remained high in the evening, and for the most part, my mood has been high as well, especially considering that at the start of the study, my energy was consistently crashing to the point where I was in bed for a good part of the afternoon.

"In the last week of the study, I still had documented one anxious evening. I cried and got pretty fired up. I still face speaking and writing about the very unpleasant situations that led to my diagnosis of Post-Traumatic Stress Disorder. I am currently involved in a pretty disturbing legal battle... Symptoms of Post-Traumatic Stress can still be triggered but attacks are not as severe and I bounce back quicker.

"Overall my mood, energy levels, ability to concentrate, and sense of wellbeing have improved since I began taking pure balanced supplements. I think they are wonderful but do want to add that I would not recommend trying to discontinue medications without the help of a therapist. When I started this trial, my brain was very dependent on the SSRIs and the clonopin. Much of the time I felt numb and without appropriate emotion. I have had to take on the task to learn a new set of coping skills as my brain heals.

"The consistent therapy combined with high-quality supplements is a package for success, but it is important to remember success still requires hard work. I have been very focused on my healing and cannot expect results to continue without continuing to put in the work. Exercise and a clean diet are very important. I have continued taking the same supplements. I feel they are worth the cost and plan to explore the benefits of the other essential oils as well, as soon as my finances allow. I am very interested in natural healing. I believe our whole society is being damaged by processed foods, medications, and imbalanced lifestyles.

"I am very happy I was given a chance to participate in this study. I hope the experiences I have documented can help encourage others who may be struggling as I have to consider taking a more natural approach to healing whenever possible."

## Weight Release

Jennifer from Oregon reports her results in only adding balanced nutrition supplements to her regular eating program for sixty days:

"Energy: Higher during the study than before. Stable. Consistent, other than when I was sick. I had much better energy levels when I was sick than I would have had before when sick.

Sleep: Nothing noticeable…however my sleep cycle was better. I have a wrist bracelet that measures activity and sleep cycles.

Weight: Lost 4.6 pounds…I lost inches from beginning to end. My clothes are a lot looser

Emotions: More consistent…Little things do not send me off, I feel much more balanced.

Appetite: Not as hungry, takes less to satisfy me, yet I still had lots of energy. Not eating out of boredom, not craving sweets! Feeling balanced! Also had regular bowel movements for the first time in my life! Normally have them every two to three days."

## Pain and Inflammation

Patricia from Oregon reports this progress on her sixty-day study period:

"Energy: I had a flare up in my immune disease that makes me exhausted all the time. I noticed I had more energy. I feel the oils were beneficial. The supplements really helped though they bothered my tummy. My pain levels went up during times of stress. I'm also on meds for this type of arthritis, and I felt the oil helped with this.

"Sleep: Some good nights, some bad nights. Neuropathy wakes me up. I have a hard time getting the oil on my feet.

"Weight: I did not weight myself, but I feel I have lost weight.

"Emotions: I felt pretty stable…even during the times of stress. I feel the products helped keep me more balanced.

"Pain: Pain levels were up and down due to activity and stress. I know I could not have done as much without the oil and supplements. I feel they helped me physically deal with what was going on.

"I was pleased to find relief from the constant pain I have. My levels started at 10 and at times were down to a 2. I actually ended at a 3-4, which was a miracle after the holiday stress. My son was in the hospital during the last two weeks of the study, which has added to the stress. Anytime I have more activity it causes me pain, too, and this was manageable with the oil."

I continue to be amazed at how many grown adults don't think that nutrition has anything to do with emotional or physical health. Here is the secret they clearly do not understand…

Your metabolism REQUIRES a wide variety of nutrients in order to digest and distribute nutrients. This is not an option but a requirement for digestive efficiency. So if ample vitamins, minerals or other micronutrients are not supplied through diet and supplements, your metabolic processes must rob the body of its own nutrient stores. Continually supplying the body with foods lacking or void of nutrients will eventually lead to serious nutritional deficiencies in different organs and body parts, which can and will create dysfunction and disorder.

Second, your entire body is a system comprised of several systems that ALL RELY on proper fuel which must come from the *macro* AND *micro*nutrient sources in order to function optimally.

The answer is simple. Having an array of balanced nutrients is important, and that can simply be done by making healthy food choices and getting a good daily balanced supplement that is completely free of synthetics, balanced like a meal, and formulated with maximum absorbency. Then you will undoubtedly experience what healthy, happy people do…a body in ORDER!

# OTHER SUPPLEMENTS THAT MIGHT BE IMPORTANT

## Enzymes

How many people do you know with digestive challenges...or should we say...how many people do you know without digestive challenges? Most people you know do have these issues even if they don't particularly know it.

Enzymes are often missing in our foods due to cooking and processing, and since most individuals don't get the amount of raw fresh vegetables and fruits that contain natural enzymes, digestive challenges may occur. Without sufficient enzymes, digestion in inhibited, undigested foods can clog your intestines and produce inflammation, which can result in a number of illnesses or disorders. A healthy digestive system is simply key to proper function of all systems in your body.

Thus a good balanced enzyme complex can be highly beneficial. Enzymes taken with meals can assist the body in the digestive process, while enzymes taken on an empty stomach between meals can break down the matter within your intestines as well as in your blood.

## Probiotics

An abundance of friendly flora is important and necessary for these reasons:

1) They keep your digestive system healthy by coating the digestive tract, creating a protective barrier that will keep harmful substances from entering the bloodstream. Strengthening the lining of the gut with probiotics is super important for preventing leaky gut and creating any deterioration along the tract.
2) They fight carcinogens and other toxic substances and help them export.
3) They assist in the digestive process by producing enzymes to help break down our foods.
4) Healthy gut flora helps protect against an overgrowth of unhealthy bacteria, as well as yeasts, viruses, and parasites.

5) They improve and enhance the overall function of our gastrointestinal tract, by strengthening the immune system.

A good live probiotic of friendly flora is a complement to your enzymes and overall digestion.

## GOALS AND SUGGESTIONS

Don't fool yourself into thinking that supplying your body with the needed balance of supplements is costly and out of your budget. CUT COSTS ELSEWHERE. Eliminate other drinks (that are so costly if you really add them all up), eliminate fast food and convenience store stopping, and make your health a priority with concentrated, balanced micronutrient sources.

Healthy happy people spend their money supporting their health with foods, supplements and activities found in nature. In doing this, they SAVE hundreds and thousands of dollars on the costs of treatment and correction…think in the Eastern mentality…and enjoy your life!

Take a sheet of paper and divide it into 3 vertical columns writing the words as such:

Goals                    Remove                    Supply

1. List your most important goals (more energy, better focus, ideal weight – be specific).
2. List the items in your diet/supplements that you need to remove to meet that goal.
3. List the items in your diet/supplements you need to supply to meet that goal.
4. Take action and do it!

# SUPPORT

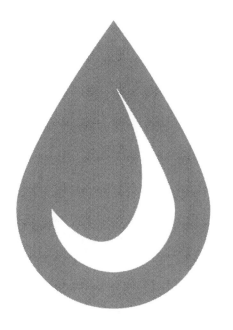

# Chapter 18

# NATURE'S PURE ESSENTIAL OILS

I got a phone call one day. It was my daughter in need, who said, "Mom, Hailey just fell and split her head open again! This is the third time in two months, and it's right on the same area of the forehead. If I take her back to the emergency room, I'm afraid they will call CPS! Is there an oil that I can use for this instead?"

"Yes," I responded. "Do you have helichrysum?"

She paused for a moment and said, "Yes." This is one of the more expensive oils due to the enormous amount of plant material needed to produce it – but it's also one of those oils that you want to have around just in case you need it. I was glad she had it.

I proceeded with the instructions to just dot the open cut directly with the helichrysum – not even a drop, just a little on her finger, then repeat another couple of times. She did that and said the cut immediately stopped bleeding, and with that and a couple more applications, it pulled the cut together and sealed it shut.

A week and a half later, they stopped by. The first thing she said when they came in the door was, "Look at Hailey's forehead. You can hardly see the cut where the helichrysum was applied, whereas you can still see the scars from the stitches."

She figured that it had cost less than $3 for the oil, while going to the emergency room she used most of her $1000 deductible both times. This time . . .

No emergency room to wait in with the trauma involved.

She was prepared ahead of time with oils needed.

She was able to act within minutes of the accident.

Spent only pennies compared to hundreds of dollars.

Effective healing without scarring.

She was so much happier with the overall results! That's the power of essential oils and the benefits that are often found!

## MODERN PHARMACEUTICALS VS. THERAPEUTIC GRADE ESSENTIAL OILS

Let's first start with Modern Pharmaceuticals, then how they compare to Therapeutic Grade Essential Oils.

Modern pharmaceuticals are highly promoted and recommended for use based on these reasons:

- big profits
- monopoly and control
- patent ability
- more control over individuals and decision making

In pharmaceuticals we find the 3 S's:

- synthetically produced in a laboratory
- designed to treat symptoms
- side effects due to their foreign nature on the body

Here is what my friend, Dr. Dominic, has to say:

"If I break a bone or get into a car accident, then there's no other country I'd rather be than right here in the U.S. We do an amazing job at trauma relief in this country, but we fail miserably when it comes to disease state management and prevention. Asking our doctors and pharmacists how to prevent XYZ disease is like asking a mechanic how to write computer code. They can't tell you because they don't know...unless they've taken it upon themselves to study it OUTSIDE of their medical curriculum. And there's very few that do. The healthcare system simply is not designed that way. It's designed to identify SYMPTOMS of a disease rather than the cause, and to treat those symptoms. Disease state management is symptom management, not prevention. To prevent the disease, YOU must take action and not rely on your doctor for the answer. That's why I use essential oils in my household. They're safe and effective in helping the body do what it is designed to do…heal from within." Dr. Dominic Hrabe, Pharm.D."

In the article "Why Essential Oils Heal and Drugs Don't", Dr. David Stewart, Ph.D., makes this statement: "…according to the U.S. Centers for Disease Control, more than 100,000 Americans die every year, not from illegal drugs, not from drug overdoses, not from over-the -counter drugs, and not from drug abuses, but from properly prescribed, properly taken prescriptions. In this country, more people die from doctor's prescriptions every ten days than were killed in the 9/11 terrorist attacks." [46] With $6.5 trillion dollars spent on healthcare annually, do you feel you (or we as a people) are getting healthier with each new-year? Are you getting the kind of care you feel is the most effective when it comes to your everyday needs?

Here is what other medical professionals have to say:

"'Every drug increases and complicates the patient's condition.' Robert Henderson, M.D.

"'What hope is there for medical science to ever become a true science when the entire structure of medical knowledge is built around the idea that there is an entity called disease which can be expelled when the right drug is found?' John H. Tilden, M.D. Author of *Impaired Health, Etiology, Hygiemic,* and *Dietetic Treatment of Appendicitis,* and other books and articles.

"'Drugs never cure disease. They merely hush the voice of nature's protest, and pull down the danger signals she erects along the pathway of transgression. Any poison taken into the system has to be reckoned with later on even though it palliates present symptoms. Pain may disappear, but the patient is left in a worse condition, though unconscious of it at the time.' Daniel. H. Kress M.D. Author of *The Cost to Society of Cigarettes: A Century of Analysis, Ulcers and Smoking,* and other books." [47]

This doesn't mean you or I should never use pharmaceuticals. They do have their place, and I am grateful for the advanced research, technology, and applications. You are always encouraged to seek professional advice as needed. But what this should mean to you is that if you want to live a healthier life you can:

1. Take better measures to prevent illness through living a healthy lifestyle to begin with: what you eat and drink is important as well as proper rest, exercise, and managing your stress.

2. EDUCATE yourself about the options when it comes to many issues you are presented with and familiarize yourself with alternatives that might be better for your body in the long run, especially in your simple day-to-day experiences.

3. Be proactive when it comes to medical care. When it is your body, or the body of one of your family members, be cautious, think long term, know what you are putting in and on your body.

Now let's look at pharmaceutical drugs and their comparison to essential oil according to Dr. David Stewart:

- Drugs create toxicity
- Drugs clog/confuse receptor sites
- Drugs depress immune system
- Drugs are unbalancing to the body
- Drugs are one dimensional
- Drugs feed misinformation into the cells to provide temporary relief without true healing
- Oils detoxify
- Oils clean receptor sites
- Oils strengthen immune system
- Oils are balancing to the body
- Oils are multi-dimensional
- Oils address the cause of disease at a cellular level, deleting misinformation and reprogramming correct information [48]

Is there a bit of a difference in how these can affect you differently?

# THE HISTORY OF ESSENTIAL OILS

Essential oils have been around for thousands of years as the most effective forms of medicine. The Egyptians were some of the first people to use aromatic essential oils extensively in medical practice, beauty treatment, food preparation, and religious ceremony. Frankincense, sandalwood, myrrh, and cinnamon were considered very valuable cargo along caravan trade routes and were sometimes exchanged for gold.

Borrowing from the Egyptians, the Greeks used essential oils in their practices of therapeutic massage and aromatherapy. The Romans also used aromatic oils to promote health and personal hygiene. Influenced by the Greeks and Romans, as well as Chinese and Indian Ayurvedic use of aromatic herbs, the Persians began to refine distillation methods for extracting essential oils from aromatic plants. Essential oil extracts were used throughout the dark ages in Europe for their anti-bacterial and fragrant properties.

In the ancient world, essential oils such as frankincense and myrrh were actually more valuable than gold and precious metals. They were common gifts given to kings and queens and hence why the three wise men brought these as a gift to the baby Jesus.

In modern times, the powerful healing properties of essential oils were rediscovered in 1937 by a French chemist, Rene-Maurice Gattefosse, who healed a badly burned hand with pure lavender essential oil. He has become known as the "father of aromatherapy" due to his extensive research and study of essential oils and their applications. Dr. Jean Valnet used therapeutic-grade essential oils to successfully treat injured soldiers during World War II. Dr. Valnet recognized the need for alternatives to medications and antibiotics, and for this reason, became proficient in application and development of many aromatherapy practices. [49]

Today much research on therapeutic-grade essential oils validates their effectiveness as a supplement for use in supporting and strengthening the body in many ways. Many individuals, families, and physicians are finding great results in their homes and workplaces. Not only are they complementing many medical settings, but they are giving people hope once again to be more in control of their health without the negative side effects.

# Chapter 19

# WHAT ARE ESSENTIAL OILS?

Essential oils are the highly concentrated, volatile, aromatic essences of plants. They contain hundreds of organic constituents and natural elements that work on many levels. They are fifty to seventy times more concentrated than the oils in dried herbs.

There are many plants found around the world that can provide quality essential oils making aromatherapy a truly global therapy. Information on the specific properties of each essential oil can be found in many books published worldwide on essential oils.

People find great benefits in using essential oils in many ways:

- Overall Wellness – In the Preface of this book was a contrast of Eastern vs. Western medicine. The Eastern medicine focus is prevention and addressing the root issues of dysfunctions. Essential oils provide great support in strengthening and providing good prevention while addressing the root causes of dysfunction at the cellular level.

- Dysfunction – Nature provides so many solutions for target support and symptom management through these tiny molecules called essential oils by soothing pain, relieving congestion, reducing stress, stimulating circulation, and providing first-aid care for many wounds, cuts, and burns. Because of this, parents are becoming educated and feel empowered to better care for their family's immediate and long-term needs.

- Body and Home Care – One's typical environment is bombarded with toxic threats every minute of the day in the form of lotions, perfumes, facial skin care, hair care, sunscreens, cleaning products, air fresheners, detergents and more. Essential oils can provide natural solutions along with alternative ingredients that support the health and well-being of your body and environment.

Aromatherapy has been used for many years for mental and emotional support and benefits. Our sense of smell is governed by the olfactory bulb which sends a signal to the limbic system in the brain. The limbic system is responsible for mood, memory, behavior, and emotions. Thus, inhaling essential oils can provide many psychological benefits, having a powerful effect upon the mind.

On the flip side, synthetic candles, air fresheners, and other toxic chemicals emit fumes which can have a powerfully negative effect on your mind, mood, memory, behavior, and emotions. Most people do not realize the harmful effects some of the chemical constituents can have on the brain. Thus removing toxic aromatics and replacing them with essential oils which promote wellness can make a huge impact upon not only your mind, but your entire physiology.

Extensive scientific research done in the past several years documents that in additional to aromatic benefits, one can also have dramatic topical and internal benefits if essential oils are 1) found in top purity and therapeutic quality based on plant quality and extraction methods, 2) applied with the best method of application, and 3) applied within the safety guidelines of dosage and repetition.

If you look at the effect upon a virus which is inner cellular, pharmaceutical antibiotics are hydrophilic – water soluble – which explains why they are not effective for viruses and only bacteria which reside outside of the cell. In contrast, essential oil are lipophilic – fat soluble – which can dissolve in fats and other lipophilic substances. Since your cells are also lipophilic this makes it easy for essential oils to penetrate the cellular wall and enhance cellular activity. In addition, this lipophilic nature makes essential oils easily absorbed by the skin and body which can make it possible for a profound healing action to take place.

When taking the role of the responsible party in applying essential oils, one must not underestimate the importance of education. Essential oils are powerful solutions found in nature. Their purity, quality, quantity, method of application, dosage, reputation and more all play an important part in the end results. So before application:

1) Choose only quality essential oils that are completely unadulterated with the highest purity and therapeutic potency. This will make a huge difference in the results you are seeking. Research the extraction methods and sourcing of your brand, as all are NOT created equal. There is no standard or regulations for the production of essential oils.
2) Become educated in essential oils and their applications.
3) Use wisdom, caution and respect for these tiny potent molecules.

See Chapter 20, The Simplicity of Essential Oils, for uses and cautions.

## Understanding Quality and Grades of Oil

There are significant differences between synthetic fragrance oils and pure, therapeutic essential oils. A growing number of products are claiming either to be essential oils or to contain essential oils. They range in price and quality and are found in skin care, cosmetics, aromatherapy, and other products. However, many of these products do not use pure essential oils and often use fragrant synthetic chemical substitutes to dilute or replace more expensive essential oil extracts. Furthermore, there are no current regulatory standards for the descriptive use of the "therapeutic grade" for products labeled as essential oils. Therefore, choose a brand of essential oils where therapeutic quality and purity are extremely important.

Essential oils with the most pure therapeutic quality can be used in three different ways for these benefits:

- aromatically – respiratory and emotional support, air purification
- topically – skin, muscle, joints, and system support
- internally – cleansing, organ support

Essential oils that can have a recommendation for internal use display the higher levels of purity and potency. Individuals or companies who shun the thought of internal use, clearly do not understand that anything applied topically or aromatically goes internally anyway. This is an important factor in choosing quality essential oils.

There are three pathways of exposure to the body which correspond to the different uses:

- respiratory system – aromatically
- skin – topically
- digestive system – internally

This is very important to understand in being able to choose the correct usage of essential oils. For example, if you are experiencing a respiratory challenge, the most likely way to use your oil is aromatically; for a sore, cut, or muscle pain, topically would usually be the obvious application; as for internal cleansing or organ support, then internally would mostly likely be your best choice.

Some essential oils can be used all three ways, for example, the onset of a virus: diffusing a protective blend of oils, dropping a few drops on the back of your tongue, and applying to the bottoms of the feet (which have the largest pores on your body for fastest circulation). You can find support and benefits all three ways.

Another one of my daughters had this experience with essential oils:

"A couple of years ago, we noticed my son, who was six, was walking a little funny. One of his feet turned in when he walked. Thinking it was just how he walked, we didn't think much of it until over some time, we saw how it was affecting the way he ran. He didn't really like us touching his feet, but one night when he was lying down, we looked at his one foot where he wasn't putting full pressure on it, and noticed a spot on the bottom of it. We weren't sure what is was but assumed it was a corn or something from rubbing in his shoe. After seeing it grow bigger over time, and noticing how uncomfortable it was for him to walk on it, we decided to take him to a podiatrist. We were surprised when he told us it was a plantar wart, and there were a couple more popping up in other areas on his foot. Because of the size of it, the doctor said it would require surgically removing it, which we would need to schedule fairly soon.

"Knowing what I had learned about oregano essential oil, and not wanting to fork the cost of surgery, I decided to give my oregano oil a chance. We started applying just a small drop on the wart a couple of times a day, and after being consistent for a couple of weeks, it completely fell out. We were totally amazed because the warts were completely gone, and the tissues healed very quickly without any pain! Our total cost? Maybe a couple of dollars – a huge savings from the proposed surgery!

"He soon began walking straight with no issues. I was even more grateful after seeing a friend of ours who had a plantar wart even smaller than our son's, had surgery to remove it, and was still in bandages and limping on it after two weeks! She said it had been a painful healing process for something she thought was so small. How grateful I am for the pure therapeutic-grade essential oils and the small miracles we've experienced! I love my oils!"

This and other stories like the following one are why I am so passionate about essential oils. My friend Jennifer writes this:

"I almost never share this story partly because even I was STUNNED by what my oils did, stunned by the power of God to heal, and because it's hard to really describe it to someone who wasn't there. In July of last year, my twelve-year old daughter got lost on her mountain bike in the mountains of Arizona behind our home. When we found her, she was in heart failure, was seizing, and had been exposed to full 115-degree sunlight for over forty minutes. After twenty-five minutes of CPR while waiting for rescue, she coded in the ambulance, and when the ambulance arrived at the hospital and wheeled her body into the hospital, the doctors pulled me aside and told me that they were sorry, but there was nothing that they could do. She did finally revive but was in a coma all day, and her core temperature didn't fall below 108 degrees for many hours, despite the cooled IVs and being packed in ice, so her brain was severely damaged and we were told again and again that she would never survive.

"When I found her in the dessert I was in a swimsuit with flip-flops and didn't have my cell phone or ANY OF MY OILS! When it became clear that doctors couldn't save my sweet daughter, I called a friend from the hospital to bring me the brain oils: frankincense, sandalwood, bergamot, and peppermint. I turned my daughter onto her side and began layering the oils down her spine every fifteen minutes, and ran the diffuser with those four oils. She was totally unresponsive to stimulation, but the first time I went down her spine with the oils, she shuddered. I began the oils around ten o'clock at night, and within an hour, she was making eye contact and muttering nonsense sounds. Soon she was talking. When she could communicate, she told me to stop the frankincense oil because it had made her body tickle when she was asleep (thus the shudder during the coma). I didn't stop. I kept going. We were told that because of the level of brain damage and the total organ failure, heart failure, and damage to her intestines, she would be hospitalized for weeks and undergo major rehabilitation and suffer permanent disability because of the traumatic brain injury. I poured a thousand dollars worth of oils down her spine that week, and on the fifth day, we walked out of the intensive care unit and headed home. The doctors were stunned.

"In the months following, doctors and neuropsychologists studied my daughter because they almost NEVER find a patient who has undergone the level of heat damage that she did and survived. We continued nightly use of the brain oils, quality supplements, enzymes, and probiotics to aid in her recovery. Immediately following the accident, she couldn't spell her name or add 2+2 and had many health issues because of the damage to her central nervous system. It's been just over a year, and she now has NO NOTICEABLE EFFECTS. You would never know that she had been literally cooked a year ago.

"I know that God brought my daughter back to life, and that he blessed me with the gift of pure oils to help support her little brain. It was so amazing to see the power of those brain oils in action."

So what's the real secret that you need to understand when it comes to essential oils?

Essential oils were created by the same creator as your body. The body mirrors plants in many of its characteristics and functions. For instance, the human genome is the basic structure of genetic information that we pass onto our children. Plant genomes are similar, as both the human genome and plant genome each contain around 25,000 genes. [50]

Human cells and plant cells each individually contain six identical active components including cell membranes, the nucleus, and mitochondria. The presence of mitochondria means both have cellular respiration for the production of energy.

Both plants and humans require nutrients for growth and life itself. As plants derive inorganic minerals from the soil to sustain itself, themselves, organic minerals that come through the plants are what sustain humans (we can't eat dirt and get the same results). The plants give off oxygen and take in carbon dioxide; humans breathe in oxygen and give off carbon dioxide. Thus plant and humans thrive through our connections in our ecosystem.

Both humans and plants have an immune system. The essential oils are specifically the plant's own defense mechanism that not only protects the plant itself from predators, but by design was created also to provide immunity and support mechanisms that would likewise benefit humans. Humans and plants communicate on a cellular level, and that's why humans find such amazing benefits and support in these concentrated, aromatic compounds because they are literal gifts to us from nature. Plants give all – benefitting humans and all mammals is the nature of their creation. Do you likewise feel love and appreciation for them and your Creator for the cellular connection that we share?

This alone is what most drives my passion for using essential oils!

# Chapter 20

# THE SIMPLICITY OF ESSENTIAL OILS

Like anything else you do, it takes education to feel comfortable in using essential oils to support and assist your body in its processes. If you are new to essential oils, and even if you are not new, read and study before you apply when you have a need or ailment.

There are several cautions and considerations in using essential oils:

- It's better to use a little bit more often than a lot at once. Essential oils are concentrated aromatic compounds, so 1-2 drops is often the dosage. However, don't think that you have to wait four hours between applications. The French Intensive Method says for the onset of an acute situation, you can use this dosage: every fifteen minutes for the first hour, every thirty minutes for the next two hours, then on the hour for the next few hours.

- Children are much smaller and depending on size, use wisdom in using 1/2 or 1/4 the amount you would as an adult.

- While most essential oils can be applied *neat* (without dilution) onto the skin, some oils are *hot* and need a carrier oil such as coconut, olive, almond, etc. with the application (fractionated coconut oil stays liquefied and is one of the best carrier oils). Children and the elderly have more sensitive skin, and you have areas on your body that are more sensitive, so be careful when using oils such as clove, oregano, peppermint, and cinnamon.

- If essential oils get into your eyes – I am so sorry – it will hurt! Rather than using water, use a carrier oil to dilute it.

- Some oils should be avoided during pregnancy to prevent the onset of labor and for other reasons. Make sure you do the research on which oils to use when pregnant.

- DO NOT create your own essential oil blends unless you are experienced in creating blends. You can diminish the effectiveness by adding them all together in a veggie capsule or roller bottle. Blending oils is an art, so if you don't know how to properly blend oils, then leave it to a company that has created their blends properly. If wanting to use more than one oil at a time, consider layering instead: drops under the tongue, topically on your skin and such. Apply one oil at a time and wait a few seconds before applying the next.

- To protect the quality and purity of essential oils, keep them out of the heat and out of the light. Essential oils found in the tombs after hundreds of years still had amazing therapeutic qualities. Good pure, therapeutic oils can and will last indefinitely if you take care of them properly, except for citrus essential oils which are cold pressed extracted. These may need to be used within two to three years for best benefits.

- If essential oils are diluted or contain contaminants, they may smell like chemicals, produce inferior results, or even be caustic.

## How Long Before You See Results?

I have seen peppermint cool and calm a headache within three to five minutes, melaleuca to soften the pain of an earache within four to five minutes as well, however, that may not always be the case. Essential oils are assisting the body with the tools needed to heal itself, so at times, it may take longer to see the results than you might hope. However, keep in mind, the long-term benefits without the side effects are usually worth it.

With a variety of essential oils available, there are beneficial applications for supporting almost any type of need – but be patient because sometimes is also takes time and a few trials to find what oils will be the most benefit to you.

I had this experience a few years ago. After one solid year of suffering with intense pain in my right shoulder and arm, I finally found relief. Not knowing what brought this on, I knew only that my arm/shoulder area just began hurting. The pain was so intense in my arm, especially at night, so I knew it was inflammation setting in. I began topically applying essential oils and blends that address pain and inflammation, and although they did help some, I continued to be in pain.

After two months, I went to my chiropractor, but as he worked on me, I yelled out in pain that put me in tears. After a few weeks of this, he sent me to get two MRIs. The results showed nothing. I decided massages were a better choice, and although this helped me tremendously, the pain during the night didn't go away. As far as essential oils, I researched more, began applying marjoram, cypress, lemongrass, peppermint, and different pain blends, but still no real improvement.

I began seeing a "soft touch" chiropractor (no popping), and for months – even though this helped me function, I was still not doing better. In the meantime, I could not lift anything (including my grandchildren, which broke my heart), and my arm became more and more immobile. After several months at the second chiropractor, I finally told him that he was helping me function, but I was not getting better, and I had to find out the problem and soon! I was tired of this! He suggested a physical therapist.

I had my first appointment, and he asked what my daily postural positions were. The culprit to my problem? Sitting at a laptop for hours during the day, shoulders hunched forward, head down. Physical therapy greatly helped me get my muscles working again, but the intense pain was still there, especially during the night.

At about month ten of this, I taught a class in California where one of the attendees picked up our essential oils reference book and randomly began to read information about white fir essential oil being helpful for: frozen shoulder, bursitis, cartilage inflammation, muscle pain, sprains, etc. I was excited – I had a new oil I could try! Once I got home, I began applying it night and morning. I felt major relief within a few days, and within a few weeks, got the full use of my arm back! There is an oil for everything! I knew it, but I had to be patient until I found it, and I was so glad when I did.

Here's another important experience that you can learn from.

My friend Sharla, who is very knowledgeable and successful in using essential oils in a variety of ways, called me one day. She had been moving a cabinet and she cut her leg mid-calf through her jeans. She took the precautions of applying several essential oils, however it still became infected.

Four weeks later, while still applying the oils faithfully, the cut was not healing so she went to her medical doctor. He recommended she get a prescription of antibiotics. As she was filling the prescription, the pharmacist mentioned the risks so she decided against taking it. Two weeks later, the cut was still not healing so she contacted me.

Here was what I thought could be the problem. She was applying great and effective essential oils for healing – however, healing wasn't the issue. Infection was, and that needed addressed. I suggested she soak her leg in Epsom salt with melaleuca essential oil three times daily. The infection was sealed under her skin with no way to escape. It needed to be opened up so the infection could come out – and even be expressed if possible. That was the focus first before the healing could occur. Soaking her leg three times was all it took. The Epsom salt and melaleuca were able to open it up and draw out the infection. And after just three soakings, the cut was no longer tender to the touch and the swelling had gone down. Now healing could take place and it did.

Now I'm no doctor, but I wonder why a medical professional wouldn't first use some common sense, instead of just recommending an antibiotic. None of us know how to handle all situations, but instead of always looking for a treatment, let's look for the cause. Here is where we will all be more successful in the final result.

# Chapter 21

# BUILDING IMMUNITY NATURALLY

There is much controversy when it comes to building immunity to certain diseases. Being raised in Western medicine myself, I have really had to do the research to find answers to this issue – and I encourage you to do likewise. You do have a choice when it comes to building your immunity, but it comes with a responsibility too. Read and ponder the following quotes…then continue to study the issues.

"All vaccines depress our immune functions. The chemicals in the vaccines depress our immune system; the virus present depresses immune function; and the foreign DNA/RNA from animal tissues depresses immunity. Studies have found that some metabolic functions were significantly reduced after vaccinations were given and did not return to normal for months. Other indicators of immune system depression included reduced lymphocyte viability, neutrophil hyper-segmentation, and reduced white cell count. We are trading a small immune depression for immunity to one disease, our only defense against all known disease for a temporary immunity against one disease, usually an innocuous childhood disease. Vaccines have been linked to AIDS and other immune-deficient disorders as well. The trade-off is not at all fair and not worth the risk." Natural News, online [51]

From *Vaccines: Are They Really Safe and Effective*, it says studies show that "many of the vaccines [do] not show that they were responsible for a decline in the incidence of the disease…Many of the vaccines also failed to show evidence of their ability to confer immunity, in fact, some studies show that the disease is more likely to be contracted by those who are vaccinated against it than by those who are left alone. Finally, many of the vaccines are unsafe. Thousands of children have been damaged by them." [52]

Dr. Boyd Haley, a biochemist at the University of Kentucky, is probably one of the world's top experts on mercury toxicity who says, "A single vaccine given to a six-pound newborn is the equivalent of giving a 180-pound adult 30 vaccinations on the same day." [53]

Vaccines, although they can have some effect, cannot build natural immunity in the body the same way that nature can or was intended to do. ANYTHING that is laboratory created with chemicals and other constituents that are foreign to the human DNA will not and cannot produce long-term health benefits. There is always that ability for a side effect, which is apparent in myriad research and information available. You must do the research on cautions and dangers of vaccines and be proactive in your choices if you feel this information resonates with you. Keep in mind that wavers are almost always available for you – all you have to do is ask for them, and then be bold in your intention based on your educated decisions.

Nature provides building immunity naturally, which is how we are meant to have increased immunity to begin with. Here are four suggestions to help build your immunity naturally. However, keep in mind that inconsistency may not bring you the results you are seeking. In other words, if you choose NOT to vaccinate, be proactive in choosing to build your immune system with nature.

1) Eat whole, eat clean. Adhere to the recommendations in the NOURISH section. Your foundation to health and wellness is your intake of foods and drink. Be choosy, eliminate processed foods, and eat whole!

2) Avoid the pollutions and those items which create toxicity in your body as discussed in the CLEANSE section and will be discussed in the PROTECT section. Cleanse your system on a regular basis as recommended, be consistent and be proactive in keeping your body free of toxic substances.

3) Support your body with concentrated whole-food supplements that are in balance and will provide whole body support and build your immunity naturally as recommended in the BUILD section. This is a fundamental part of health in this period of time to offset nutritional deficiencies – it's not just an option.

4) Choose nature's medicines: herbals and essential oils. In my past thirty years, I've definitely seen the most effective results with the purest, therapeutic-grade essential oils found. And the real beauty of oils is that you can even take them on a daily basis to continually strengthen and support your immune system naturally and effectively.

That said, this information is not meant to diagnose, treat, prevent, prescribe, or take the place of your doctor's advice. It is only intended for educational purposes. Any decision you make for your health and your family's health must accompany education, common sense, and a responsibility. I strongly caution you to be educated and seek professional advice as needed. In doing so, choose a physician who is willing to support your intentions and desires. You are hiring him or her, so make sure he or she is supporting your lifestyle choices. And you can do any physician a favor by educating them with information and results you find positive from nature.

The goal is to work together as a community of people through education and application. I believe that most physicians in our medical community are there because they truly desire to make a difference, and they often too are frustrated with the results due to their educated recommendations. Show them kindness and understanding, and be willing to share good information with them in a positive way. Together we can and will all make a difference for the better.

## GOALS AND SUGGESTIONS

1. Take time out today, tomorrow or within the next few days to find a quiet spot in nature and just sit and ponder for a long period of time if possible. Listen to the sounds of nature, rub your hands through the grass (unless it's in a park that is most likely sprayed with chemicals), touch the flowers and plants, smell them, watch the

trees blow in the wind, and remember this was all created for you by a God who loves you. It's part of who you are and should be. Realize that what is found in nature is intended to support you, strengthen you, and provide tools that your body needs and ultimately desires. Now take a notepad and write down the things you are grateful for.

2. Be at peace as you begin making changes in your diet and these other lifestyle choices. You are a strong human being and can choose healthier options simply. FOCUS on healthy, happy peoples' lifestyle choices. Make them your own. Love, love, love good foods, good pure water, good healthy supplements, and pure essential oils that have the ability to support healthy lifestyle habits. Take time right now to write a paragraph on why this is important for your long-term success. Then share it with a spouse or friend so they can help keep you accountable for that success

# STRENGTHEN

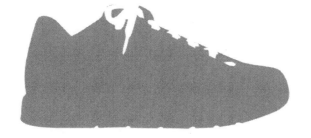

# Chapter 22

# REGULAR EXERCISE

Many of you may be able to relate with my friend Holly's story:

"Back in 2009, I began struggling with severe and constant muscle cramps, raw nerves, skin sensitivities, mood swings, insomnia, and cellular pain 24/7. This was debilitating enough to keep me bedridden for much of my days. For the most part, I felt it was accelerated by stress due to the adoption of our three children from another country, the passing away of my mom, and other stressful factors that were also possible contributors. This led me into self-medicating myself with foods, gaining weight, and more pain. I went to my doctor, who prescribed sleeping pills, pain relievers, anti-depressants, but none of those were helping me. I didn't really understand much about what was creating my stress or my pain, but I did know I needed to do something different, and I needed to lose weight.

"I attended a three-day Women's Health Retreat, began taking classes, and was discovering the benefits of nutrition and living a healthier life, but I didn't have the willpower to make the changes that would create a difference for me in reducing my stress, my pain, or my weight. But little by little, I kept learning.

"In 2011, I began learning about essential oils, so I started with lemon grass and clove, which helped somewhat helped lesson my pain. I liked the essential oils, but not until I finally gave in and started a balanced nutritional supplement and full-on cleansing program was I able to get rid of my sugar cravings. I learned that candida was a huge contributor to not only my pain, but also my stress and my weight. I was able to cleanse the candida, but I still didn't lose any weight. I knew that sugar was a huge problem and contributor, and I didn't consistently exercise because my hip would hurt, and I would stop.

"A year ago, I was introduced to a fitness program through one of my friends in Colorado who was finding success, and I decided to learn more. It sounded like fun, there was a social aspect of it, people were having success, and there was competition with cash awards that piqued my interest. We as a family – including my husband and teenage boys – decide to follow this program faithfully for ninety days. Daily, there were 100 points possible per person, which had to be reported by each of us daily for doing the full exercise program, eating good choices of foods, taking balanced supplements, drinking plenty of water that included essential oils for cleansing out the toxicity, as well as other simple daily challenges. It was that commitment, that accountability that helped us find success and kept us on track, which really paid off, literally, as we were one of the grand prize winners of the competition.

"But the best part of it all was that I finally truly learned what being healthy means. Choosing to eat very clean foods was a huge part of the program so I pulled out my healthy recipe books, got rid of all the white sugar, substituted chocolate with carob, and I learned that I could still enjoy life by eating healthy. For Thanksgiving Day, we made a new family tradition by making only healthier choices of foods: pumpkin pie, sweet potatoes etc., all in healthier forms. Because our taste buds had changed over those first sixty days, not only were these foods yummy, it was simple to do, and we all enjoyed the way we felt.

"As far as my weight, I started at 153 and went down to 127, which is a weight that I feel good at and have been able to maintain. The workouts helped to firm my body, but it was the entire program of eating good food, taking my supplements, the water, the oils and all the rest that did it for me. In the process – and it is a process – my pain changed from cellular pain to muscular pain (by working out). Even though there are great essential oils and blends that are very effective for pain – cellular pain is different. Addressing it internally by drinking water and adding the cleansing oils such as lemon, grapefruit, peppermint, cinnamon, and more, this is what made the biggest difference, along with omitting inflammatory foods such as white sugar and white flour. Energy wise, I no longer experienced afternoon fatigue. I felt excited to be alive. This made a huge difference in affecting my emotional state as well. Even though I still have several potential stress factors in my life with our adopted children, I no longer feel the need to turn to unhealthy foods or medications. I found that it is so much easier to deal with stressful situations when I am doing all the right things: eating clean, wholesome foods, exercising, drinking water, taking essential oils. When my emotional state is strengthened, I have more love and intimacy. We do better as a couple and as a family when we have common goals. We are more one because we are focused on the same thing. Once I got through the ninety days and got those results, I wanted to maintain how I felt and have continued to abide by this program because I love how I feel physically and emotionally.

"I love my medical doctor. He is a great guy, and the things he offered me were what he learned and understood might be helpful for me; however, I needed a different chemistry for my body. This is a journey, and I'm still working to improve and make it better – but I've truly come to understand it is lifestyle that works simply because of how nature's chemistry works for my body."

What's the real secret to weight release? Eat right and exercise more! It's not rocket science. It's common sense! And you get all the other physical and emotional benefits that go along with it, just as Holly shared!

## EXERCISE

Every day you consume calories through the foods you eat, and because of this, you must burn the calories you are consuming, which in turn will strengthen your organs, muscles, bones, and all your body systems. Exercise is not an option for healthy, happy people. Just like eating, it's part of one's daily activities.

Daily physical exercise can provide many benefits to you such as:

- sleeping more soundly
- thinking more clearly and more logically
- feeling more energetic throughout the day
- having a toner system
- losing weight naturally
- having organs, muscles, and bones working more efficiently

- reducing your stress naturally
- aging more gracefully
- accomplishing more each and every day!

One particular study showed a scenario that can be typical for women who eat fairly well yet don't exercise as they age:

1. Age 20 – 120 lbs. size 8
2. Age 40 – 120 lbs. size 10
3. Age 60 – 120 lbs. size 12

Even though I cannot document the source of this study, let's discuss why this might be a true scenario.

1) Fat weight takes up more space than muscle weight. Without exercise, you lose muscle weight, and it is replaced with fat weight which can increase your size without increasing your weight.

2) People naturally tend to lose muscle and gain fat as they age because they are typically less active!

Although a complete workout should include four components, you will find best results by varying your daily workout routines that include these, such as this example:

- Monday: complete workout
- Tuesday: mini-trampoline workout
- Wednesday: complete workout
- Thursday: mountain biking or swimming session
- Friday: complete workout
- Saturday: hiking or trail brisk walking
- Sunday: give your body a day off

## Four Components of a Complete Workout

Always drink a large glass of water before you work out to hydrate yourself. If you want to increase fat burning, you can add one to two drops of grapefruit or lemon essential oil.

1. **Stretching:** Flexing and stretching keeps your body limber, giving your muscles the ability to move over a wide range without stiffness. Stretching before any workout will most often prevent tearing or staining your muscles. Include deep breaths and stretch (not bounce) your arms, neck, torso, legs, and thighs for several minutes before and after any workout. Yoga or even applied yoga techniques are very effective.

2. **Muscular Fitness or Strength Training:** Anything that can create muscle resistance is good strength training: lifting sand or metal weights, using resistance bands, pushups/pull ups are all examples. You don't need a gym membership to accomplish this, but you do need a plan and the right tools to help you be consistent. Strength training improves your overall endurance, helps you perform better at your daily tasks, primes your body for burning fat throughout the day (which is why a good workout in the morning is more advantageous), and it improves bone density. It is not necessary to do strength training every day.

3. **Aerobic Fitness:** Aerobic means "with oxygen" which is any exercise which causes you to breathe harder and increase your heart beat. Oxygen is needed not just in your lungs but on a cellular level, so as you run, brisk walk, swim, jump on a trampoline, dance, you are exercising your cardiovascular system, increasing oxygen on a cellular level, strengthening your organs, improving your body's endurance and ability to think more clearly, plus burning fat and calories in the process. A twenty-minute jog / workout, or thirty- to forty-five-minute brisk walk/hike daily is the ideal.

4. **Cool Down:** Always end your workout – whether complete workout, biking, etc. – by walking at a medium pace then stretching out again for a few minutes to allow your heart rate to come down slowly and muscles to stretch.

**One Important Tip:** If you are doing a home workout, find a time and place with minimal distractions. You will find greater success by following a workout video, by listening to X number of songs, by having an outline and setting a timer, for example, than if these are not in place.

Alicia shares her success story...

"I have three children. I lost the "baby" weight from my first before her first birthday. So I thought that was the norm. After my second, even though I gained the same amount of weight as my first, I could not lose it. I would lose some and then gain it back. I pretty much maintained my weight at 145-150 pounds. After my third, I was able to make it back to the 145-150 range, but no less. I was wearing size 11/12 jeans. I joined a gym for over two years. I did enjoy going and working out in the classes. I felt good after a workout. But I was not seeing any results. After seeing the results of my aunt and uncle I decided to put my gym membership on hold just to try out this 90-day challenge.

"I started a fitness challenge group in January with balanced nutritional supplements, the GI Cleanse, and an essential oil metabolic blend to help me. I was amazed that I did not experience any major cravings! I was able to cut out sugar, processed foods, and unhealthy carbs. I began to search for a variety of recipes to make with my "clean" food options and started putting the good ones into a notebook to turn to on a regular basis.

"I did the workout five days a week. I did the daily challenges. I learned to make better food choices that my family actually liked. I found that the most difficult time to stick to the "clean" food was during menstruation. I'm still trying to overcome that time. But it's been two months, and I've lost twelve pounds and plan to lose about eight more. I wear size 8/9 jeans now. I feel stronger and healthier, and the best thing is that my children and husband are doing this along with me.

"They are learning to make wise food choices and the importance of exercise. I love that I am doing this for them just as much as for me. Another plus is that I have extra money from canceling my gym membership! I love this new lifestyle! Yeah!"

# Chapter 23

# SPEEDING UP YOUR METABOLISM

Metabolism is the process by which your body burns calories to fuel its daily functions. Whether you are asleep or awake, your metabolism is always working. While the process is rather simple, you may be sabotaging your metabolism because you don't understand how to harness this ability to give you more energy and burn more fat.

Here are some specific ways to speed up your metabolism:

1. Follow a good daily exercise program. Exercising first thing in the morning rather than later in the day is to your advantage. Not only will you expend large amounts of energy during the times you exercise, but your metabolism continues to work all day as your muscles recover and rebuild, which contributes to more calorie and fat burning. In the morning, your body doesn't have any carbohydrates as energy to use, so you have a great opportunity to *burn fat instead of carbs*. ALWAYS drink a large glass of water prior, and don't eat a full breakfast (though a half of an apple or other fruit is important for fuel) before you exercise because you'll just give your body the carbohydrates as a source of energy instead of the body fat that you want to burn for energy.

2. You can still work out later in the day, but understand that when you go to sleep, your metabolism will slow down, and you'll miss out on all the extra fat that you can burn during the day if you had exercised first thing in the morning. When you sleep, your metabolic rate is always at its slowest.

3. What you eat for breakfast will enhance your metabolism or sabotage it, depending on your choices of foods. High carbs and high fats will sabotage it, and a great Sunrise Smoothie (see recipe in Chapter 30), eggs or other lean protein will enhance it.

4. Eating five smaller meals a day (or three medium meals and two healthy snacks) rather than two or three large meals will benefit you. You will have enough energy throughout the day, and you will more likely be free of any headaches, hunger pangs, or mood swings that you get when you are famished. Also, when eating, fill a small plate, and establish the rules for yourself – *no second helpings,* and stop eating when full!

5. All of your calories come from the food you eat. Fast foods and processed boxed meals that are high in sugar, saturated fats, artificial sweeteners, and low in water and fiber require little digestion, and *actually slow down digestion,* which causes those calories to turn immediately into adipose or fat tissue. So what you eat definitely influences your metabolism and mood, making you either sluggish or energetic.

6. *Foods that are high in nutrition and fiber will promote speeding up your metabolic rate* as a healthier digestion takes place. Wholesome foods that are high in nutritional value take more processing power to extract all those vital nutrients the body needs to run at peak efficiency. The body is actually *burning large amounts of calories just to digest these foods,* particularly if they are high in fiber. It is often noted that some foods may even have negative calories, meaning it actually takes more caloric energy to digest them than they themselves provide. Many fruits and vegetables especially fall into this category because of their high fiber content. Improving digestion this way also strengthens the liver, kidneys, and lungs, all of which facilitate a healthier metabolism.

7. Do not skip meals, especially breakfast. Eating breakfast not only can eliminate the cravings you might have later on, but you will have more energy in the morning, and can lessen your stress levels. Eating erratically signals the body to burn slower and conserve fat. This is why one who skips meals can have a harder time burning fat on only 1,200 calories a day. Having smaller meals and snacks that are higher in nutrition throughout the day is so much better.

8. Eat some kind of a protein AND some live, raw food with each meal or snack. Protein will keep you satisfied longer and will help eliminate hunger cravings, while raw foods provide better digestion and more nutrition.

9. Eat meals that include a large portion of vegetables – mostly raw, some lightly steamed if desired. Vegetables are high in vitamins, minerals and fiber and low in calories. Eat one or two raw fruits daily too.

10. Eat healthy sources of fats (olive oil, coconut oil, omega-3 oils, avocados, seeds and nuts) as they promote longer-lasting, stable energy levels, and offer the essential fats and proteins we need for better digestion and muscle building.

11. Drinking three to four quarts of water each day will create better digestion (better emptying of the stomach and intestines, less gas, bloating, constipation) and a flatter tummy. Staying hydrated also reduces headaches and fights fatigue. However, you don't want to dilute and water-log the stomach acids during your digestive process, so drink well upon rising and between meals, and only a small amount with meals as needed.

12. Add essential oils to your water to provide additional endurance, accelerate cleansing, and increase fat burning: lemon, grapefruit, cinnamon, peppermint and ginger are good choices for increasing cleansing, burning fat, building endurance and raising your metabolism.

13. Don't go "on a diet" if you need to shed some pounds...instead go on a CLEANSE! Go back to the CLEANSE section, follow the Cleansing program, and Chapter 29, Cleansing Diet: Creating Meal Plans. Doing this will get your body back in order and weight release will come naturally.

As your metabolism increases, you'll feel more energetic and lighter. As your digestion improves, the stomach empties more regularly, and you feel thinner in the waistline and less full in the chest. Once you have a faster metabolism, you will have fewer food cravings and feel more in control of your eating.

## INCORPORATE ACTIVE SEGMENTS THROUGHOUT YOUR DAY

There are several ways to increase your exercise and activities throughout the day – just keep these things in mind:

- Brisk walk or bike to a neighbor, neighborhood market, to your children's school, etc. instead of driving.
- When shopping, park your car way out in the parking lots. Walk briskly to the store, through the malls, etc. See the distance as your advantage!
- Spend your computer time standing instead of sitting. Do leg lifts, squats, etc. to break up the monotony.
- Sit on an exercise ball when you do sit.
- Spend your television time stretching, weight lifting, or jumping on a trampoline.
- You can also spend your reading time on a stationary bicycle!
- Enjoy the great outdoors – in the park, in your garden, on a hike, even just walking in a neighborhood! Get outdoors more – but stay away from inhaling traffic exhaustion!
- Use stairs over elevators or escalators if they are available – let people stare all they want!

Just look for opportunities to work your body just a little bit more in what you do.

### FOR THE ATHLETE

Essential oils can greatly enhance your workout with greater endurance and more efficiency. Essential oils pass through the cell walls quickly, they are absorbed almost instantly and can be immediately used by your body. This is why they can be so effective for athletes. Additionally, essential oils can enhance physical therapy and other recovery tactics and can support a quicker recovery. Essential oils can be administered by one of three methods: diffused *aromatically*, applied *topically*, or taken *internally* as dietary supplements.

Here are several suggestions that can be very beneficial:

## Pre Workout

For increased endurance: Apply 1-2 drops peppermint essential oil or respiratory essential oil blend on the chest, back of the neck, or bottoms of the feet to open the airways. Peppermint increases oxygen, reduces pain, assists digestion too.

To warm your muscles and increase circulation: Apply a few drops of a massage essential oil blend including (or single essential oils): cypress for circulation, marjoram for muscles, and peppermint for increased energy. You can dilute by following with fractionated coconut oil or combining with oils in palm of hand before applying.

Hydrate and raise your metabolism: Hydrate thoroughly 15-20 minutes before workout with a large glass of water which includes a few drops of lemon or grapefruit essential oil, or a metabolic essential oil blend. These oils are cleansing, and stress reducing.

If outdoors: Apply lavender essential oil with fractionated coconut oil or Ultimate Skin Protection Oil (see Chapter 32) to skin that will be exposed to the sun. Lavender is soothing and nourishing.

## During Workout

Increase alertness and focus: Diffuse peppermint and orange essential oils (2-3 drops of each in diffuser with water). Or layer each oil on chest topically if needed. Orange is stress reducing and uplifting, while peppermint is invigorating.

Boost metabolism and increase energy: Sip water periodically (from glass water bottle only) which includes a few drops of lemon or grapefruit essential oil, or a metabolic essential oil blend (including cinnamon, ginger, peppermint, lemon and more). A metabolic blend added to your water throughout the day additionally will continue to help raise your metabolism, curb your appetite, balance your blood sugar, and increase your energy.

Endurance: Applying peppermint essential oil topically to chest or inhaling during a long and tiring training session will help you feel refreshed and ready for more.

## Post Workout

Address challenged muscles: Apply a massage essential oils blend or pain blend to support and strengthen these areas, and reduce inflammation.

Bring balance: Apply sandalwood essential or a balancing essential oil blend (including spruce, frankincense, blue tansy and more) to the balls of feet and top of spine for increased physical and emotional support, and reduced stress.

If outdoors: Again follow up with applying lavender essential oil with fractionated coconut oil or Ultimate Skin Protection Oil (Chapter 32) to skin exposed to the sun.

Lavender is excellent for soothing burns and protecting your skin, as well as beneficial for sores, scrapes, cuts.

Hydrate thoroughly: After any workout, make sure you are drinking plenty of water (not other liquid pollutions) which includes a few drops of lemon or grapefruit essential oil, or a metabolic essential oil blend. These oils are cleansing, and stress reducing.

Would you like to know how to be more successful at exercising? Here is an important secret that you will want to know.

Simply put, it's really not a mind over matter thing – you and many others have tried that right? You want to exercise, you set a goal, you want to be more fit, but the truth of the matter is that you most often don't FEEL like it. Why don't you feel like it?

FUEL! If you don't earnestly feel like exercising and love doing it, it's because of the fuel you give your body. Remember what we learned in Chapter 16 with Barbara Reed Stitt's studies…you have to feed the brain, and the physical will follow. Until you GET IT when it comes to the fuel you feed your body, you won't FEEL like exercising and you probably won't find the success you desire. Are you ready to learn what specifically you need to do in addition to following those steps to increasing your metabolism? Here it is:

EAT SNACKS! Really? This will either make you or break you so read carefully and follow specifically!

When you skip meals or only eat two or three large meals in a day, you are usually so famished that you overeat and gorge yourself on unhealthy foods. It's the nature of your system – you are starving and this puts your body in fat-storing mode! Your body is not quite sure when it's going to get its next meal so it holds on to your fat for energy storage.

Snacking will give your body permission to "let it go" because more will be coming soon, not to worry. Your organs work happily in harmony with your body and with less stress. And just so you know – what creates stress more than anything is lack of nutrients and too much toxicity to keep up with the demand – remember Holly's story. So how about learn how to reverse this by giving your body more nutrients in a timely manner so your metabolism is in fat-burning mode instead of fat-storing mode. Get it?

Again, your choice of snacks is what will make you or break you. Discard all cookies, chips, candies, pastries, soft drinks, other drinks of any kind, and remove these from your shopping list permanently. Don't consider breads either. You can learn to create simple snacks that will empower you and energize your mind so that your body responds with "I want to go and exercise!" Here are some examples for one person for one snack time (mid-morning or mid-afternoon):

- 1 sliced apple and 1 tablespoon raw almond butter
- 2 stalks celery or 1 large carrot (cut up) plus 1 tablespoon raw almond butter
- 1 apple, 1 pear, or 1/2 fresh blueberries or other berries plus a few raw almonds (soaked almonds are preferred for best digestion)
- 1 cup leftover Sunrise Smoothie
- 2 1-inch squares Energy Bars or Healthy Fudge plus half an apple or stalk of celery
- 1 whole orange or grapefruit (peel it like an orange) plus a 1-inch square Energy Bars or Healthy Fudge
- veggie sticks (red peppers, celery, carrots, etc.) with a rounded tablespoon of Hummus
- small chunk of Cinnamon Trio (golf ball size) on occasion

See Chapter 30 for all recipes mentioned.

You got it – the secret to exercising more is empowering your body emotionally and physically with nutritious foods to begin with and healthy snacks to sustain and support increased metabolism and energy. Your body craves nutrition, and that is often why you may overeat because your body is not yet satisfied, so as you feed your body nutritious foods, you will naturally eat less at meal time as you eat these satisfying health snacks. These are all healthy foods that will nourish you and fill your body's reserves that have been depleted.

In addition, make sure to also include…have you read this yet…lots of pure water with essential oils in it to increase your cleansing action as well. This in conjunction puts your body in healthy happy harmony – YES!

## GOALS AND SUGGESTIONS

1. Invite your spouse or friend(s) to be your workout partner(s). Schedule your daily exercise time and routine, make it fun and a time of the day you look forward to. Share with them what you are learning, and even buy them this book so they can learn along with you (don't give it to them – you'll need it to refer to yourself).

2. As you look in the mirror, see a child of God who has value. Love your body as the housing of your spirit. Treat it with great respect by eating right, exercising regularly, and doing those things that will bring honor to your Creator. He loves you. Show him how you love this body gift he has given you by treating YOU right.

# PROTECT

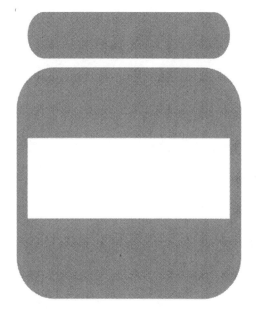

# Chapter 24

# HOW TOXIC ARE YOUR HOME CLEANERS?

We had a Chihuahua named Kizzy for over 10 years. She became part of the family like many animals do and we really loved this little dog. A few months past her tenth birthday, we noticed a tumorous growth at her groin. We did what we could do with oils and found no success so we took her into the vet to check her out. The vet suggested surgery, hospitalization, the whole nine yards with over $5000 in costs, which we considered. She did explain the risks at her age and her size (under 7 lbs.). But when I took her back in for another checkup, I asked the vet point blank, "What are her chances of living a normal life after surgery even if all goes well?" She tried to answer but honestly admitted that she didn't give her much hope for a normal life even if she survived.

We were sad but decided to let her live out her life naturally which was tough, but we felt it was the right thing to do. There were many tender moments as we watched her go downhill very fast – it only took about five months in all. Towards the end, she couldn't walk at all, we had to take her out and hold her up to eliminate. Because she was dying it was a most horrid smell that she was expelling. There were several times when she tried to get out of her bed on her own and ended up spewing all over the carpet. It was an awful smell and it discolored the carpet!

Well, I went and got out the carpet shampoo spot cleaner, then the pet cleaners for carpet – but nothing worked. The smell and the discoloration were still there – then I remembered lemon essential oil. I had used it before with great success, but not sure why I didn't think of that first. I dropped several drops all over the areas and took a hot wet cloth and scrubbed it lightly. Wow! The stains and smell both came out completely! I could hardly believe how well it worked in spite of how bad it was…Chemical cleaners could NOT come close to cleaning those spots! Thanks to my lemon essential oil that saved the day. I've looked several times since then to find any trace of discoloration on that carpet and none is to be found!

To keep a home and family clean requires a variety of soaps, detergents, bleach, softeners, bathroom cleaners, deodorizers, glass cleaners, drain and oven cleaners at one time or another. However, household cleaners are some of the most toxic substances that we encounter each day. Organic Consumers Association reports that, "In 2000, cleaning products were responsible for nearly 10% of all toxic exposures reported to U.S. Poison Control Centers, accounting for 206,636 calls. Of these, 120,434 exposures involved children under six, who can swallow or spill cleaners stored or left open inside the home." [54]

It was noted in another study that "over a 15-year period, women who cleaned their own homes had a 54% higher death rate from cancer than women who did not." [55] So women, that should give you two choices if you want to lower your cancer risk:

1. don't clean your home, or
2. don't clean your home with chemical cleaners.

Some cleaners might cause minor skin or respiratory irritations, while others may be dangerously poisonous and be carcinogenic. The most dangerous of cleaners are drain cleaners, toilet bowl cleaners and oven cleaners which can cause harm when inhaled, but also long-term illnesses as well. Ingredients such as: chlorine bleach, ammonia, formaldehyde, lye and more are specific health hazards and should be avoided as much as possible.

Some of the ingredients in detergents are known to be carcinogens and hormone disruptors:

- sudsing agents diethanolamie (DEA) and triethanolamine (TEA)…these two are often combined with nitrites (and often undisclosed) that form nitrosamines – carcinogens that readily penetrate the skin

- 1,4-dioxane, made with ethoxylated alcohols
- butyl cellosolve (also known as ethylene glycol monobutyl ether), which may cause damage to the brain and nervous system
- alkylphenol ethoxylates (APEs) known as a hormone disruptor, shown to mimic hormone estrogen
- APE, p-nonylphenol, has caused estrogen-sensitive breast cancer cells [56]

Surprisingly many fragrances are toxic too (air fresheners, hand soap, detergents, perfumes), in fact, The National Institute of Occupational Safety and Health found that one-third of the substances used in fragrances are toxic. However, companies aren't required to list their ingredients since some of them may be trade secrets, so they are merely labeled "fragrance." [57]

Another concern that is often overlooked: "In a May 2002 study of contaminants in stream water samples across the country, the U.S. Geological Survey found persistent detergent metabolites in 69% of streams tested. Sixty-six percent contained disinfectants." [58] That could mean that playing in the streams, rivers, and lakes may mean playing in contaminated water, still an additional threat.

Once consumers use a variety of toxic cleaning products and other contaminants, they go down the drain, into the sewers, then into the lakes, rivers and oceans that continue to create ongoing threats to plants and animal life through the waterways. So choosing non-toxic cleaners will benefit you in two ways:

- lessoning the direct threat of toxicity onto your skin
- lessoning the indirect threat of toxicity in your food by way of plants and animals through our water systems

Solvents such as gasoline, thinners, polish remover, and degreasers are another area of toxic substances to avoid in addition to paints, glues, alcohol perfumes, alcoholic beverages, etc. which are all toxic to the body. Solvents are highly volatile. We inhale the fumes, and they can quickly absorb into the body. Plus, if a solvent such as fingernail polish remover can dissolve something as hard as nail polish, what else might it be doing to your sensitive, absorbent skin? Think about this!

Here are some suggestions of what you can do about it:

- Avoid chemical cleaners and aerosols as much as possible – dispose of those you have.
- When cleaning of any kind, if using chemical cleaners (even if washing dishes) use rubber gloves.
- When using paints and any chemical cleaners, use rubber gloves, cover your body with clothing, wear a face mask and goggles, keep the air flowing with good ventilation with open windows and a fan.
- Consider making many of your home cleaners. They are super simple to make, only contain a few simple ingredients, and are very inexpensive in comparison to your many toxic cleaners available for purchase. See Chapter 31 for recipes.

Again, it's all about choices and better insignificant choices can make a huge difference in your health and the health of those around you!

# Chapter 25

# HOW TOXIC
# ARE YOUR FOODS?

With all the agencies in place regulating farming practices, you would think that the foods you purchase would be safe for consumption. However, follow along and see if you still agree that they are:

"As pathogens, heavy metals, and toxic chemicals from things like cleaning products and personal care products are stripped from the water, they're left behind in the human sewage waste sludge. Too toxic to incinerate, landfill, or dump at sea, the regulatory framework changed to allow this human sewage sludge to be used as a fertilizer on food crops. About 75 percent of all of the toxic sewage sludge produced in the United States winds up on farmland, potentially polluting the land with flame retardants, medical waste, and hard-to-kill bacteria and viruses." [59]

In addition, many pesticides, insecticides, fungicides, herbicides and rodenticides have carcinogenic qualities that can cause harm to the development of children. Many of these contain heavy metals such as mercury, cadmium, and lead which have been associated with a variety of types of cancer and children's developmental and behavioral issues.

Traditional farming practices here in the U.S. today, and the increased amount of chemicals have created many damaging effects in the human body, which can lead to a host of health issues that are often fatal. Although there are many foods tested that do not show the presence of pesticides, however, 93 percent of Americans tested by the CDC had metabolites of chlorpyrifos — a neurotoxic insecticide — in their urine. Though this family of pesticides was banned from home use because of its risk factors for children being linked to ADHD [60], approximately 10 million pounds of this insecticide are still being used annually in U.S. agriculture. [61]

Some of the known possible threats of pesticides and other chemicals mentioned in agricultural practices can include: digestive issues, sleep issues, lack of energy and focus, birth defects, brain damage, tumors, twitching, spasms, and more.

Again, consider the main goal of each of these is to "kill" smaller organisms, but the accumulative effect is what creates the danger especially in children, but to any human beings who consume them. So if you are eating foods grown traditionally, then you are most likely consuming these chemicals in abundance in fast foods, restaurants and grocery stores, which can pose potential threats to your overall health.

Another potential health threat is the common practice of feeding animals growth hormones for quick growth. These artificial hormones have been shown to create harmful effects for the animals as well as humans who consume them. By consuming meat and milk products, you are consuming these artificial growth hormones which can lead to dysfunction in human hormones, and can be linked to the development of many fatal diseases. Additionally, because manure is used in many farming practices and especially in home gardens, beware and avoid any feed lot manures from your local nurseries, as well as the foods that are produced by them.

To avoid the many chemical pesticides, insecticides, etc., and artificial growth hormones, here is what you can do:

- Shop for organically grown foods when at all possible – this is a huge advantage.
- Restrict eating out to times only when necessary.
- Avoid purchasing meats, milk products, mainstream market foods, and manures for gardening that most likely contain artificial growth hormones.
- Grow many of your foods organically, if possible, and use organic fertilizers and soils.
- Be choosy and intentional in the foods you regularly consume.
- Always wash your produce thoroughly to remove any toxic chemical residues (see recipe in Chapter 31).

## Buying Organic Foods

Organic foods are those produced using environmentally sound methods that do not involve modern synthetic inputs such as pesticides, chemical fertilizers, sewage sludge, bioengineering, ionizing radiation, and cannot be genetically modified (GMO). Meats are grown without antibiotics, growth hormones, and GMO foods. Organic foods are not treated with industrial solvents, waxes, colors, chemical food additives or such. [62]

For the vast majority of human history, agriculture can be described as "organic". Only during the 20th century was a large supply of new synthetic chemicals introduced to the food supply. The organic farming movement arose in the 1940s in response to the industrialization of agriculture known as the Green Revolution.

Organic food production is a heavily regulated industry, distinct from private gardening. Currently, the European Union, the United States, Canada, Japan, and many other countries require producers to obtain special certification in order to market food as "organic" within their borders. Some certifications allow some chemicals and pesticides to be used, so consumers should be aware of the standards for qualifying as "organic" in their respective locales. In the context of these regulations, "organic food" is food made in a way that complies with organic standards set by national governments and international organizations.

In the United States, organic production is a system that is managed in accordance with the Organic Foods Production Act (OFPA) of 1990, which includes integrating cultural, biological, and mechanical practices that foster cycling of resources, promoting ecological balance, and conserving biodiversity. Before foods can be labeled USDA Organic, they must pass those standards.

Organic foods are obviously going to have a higher price tag, but if you weigh out the advantages, you are certainly not paying more in the long run. You are what you eat. Are your health and your body worth it? You decide!

## The Dirty Dozen

Each year, Environmental Working Group (www.ewg.org) puts out a Dirty Dozen list of the highest pesticide load produce. These are the foods they recommend to especially avoid grown conventionally, and chose ONLY ORGANICS:

- apples
- peaches
- nectarines
- strawberries
- grapes
- celery
- spinach
- sweet bell peppers
- cucumbers
- cherry tomatoes
- snap peas (imported)
- potatoes
- hot peppers
- blueberries
- lettuce

However, produce like avocados, bananas, asparagus, onions, mangos, and papaya are low on the list and are not as important to buy organically. Be aware, be choosy.

# Chapter 26

# HOW TOXIC ARE YOUR SKIN CARE, BODY CARE, HAIR CARE, AND MORE?

Jerah from Georgia sent me her story, "I have to tell you my story. There are so many bugs and insects out here in Georgia its crazy!!! I let the kids go out in the backyard, and they were only out there for maybe fifteen minutes before they came inside covered in bug bites!! The next evening we were going out to watch fireworks, July 3, so I decided to use my oils...the kids had not one bug bite!! And the following day, July 4th, we went to a church member's house who lives on a huge lake. You could smell the bug spray people had caked on, but I brought my essential oil blend for insects and used that instead. While everyone else was fending off the massive mosquitos, we were enjoying the fireworks and friends. Now I carry it with me where ever I go. In a 2 oz. glass spritzer bottle, I add about 10 drops of an essential oil repellent blend and fill it with water. Whenever we go out I 'mist' the kids! I love it! I love seeing the oils work so well."

The amount of toxic chemicals found in all types of skin care products is unbelievable, and they don't even work as well as what you find in pure essential oils.

Do you know what you are putting on your skin?

As we've already discussed in previous chapters, your skin is the largest organ on your body. It protects your organs, it moves nutrients and wastes through our blood and lymph, and this is an important reason to make sure you protect your skin by applying toxic- free, nourishing, and health-

153

promoting skin care, body care, hair care, cosmetics and any form of self-care products that address the skin.

You and I know that we don't necessarily want everything regulated in this country, but you need to clearly understand that in the skin care and cosmetic industry, no one is required to test many of the products you may be using on your skin. You don't know if they have potential harmful agents that could create long-term side effects. Many available products on the market are linked to birth defects, infertility, other health challenges, and sometimes even life-threatening effects. Since your skin easily absorbs anything you apply on it, it's important to be aware of the possible dangers.

As mentioned earlier, it's the accumulative effect that is the biggest concern. With women using up to fifty different toxic products on a daily basis (hair care, skin care, body care, cleaning products, sunscreens, etc.), it makes sense that you might actually be acquiring more toxic chemicals through your skin than you would through what you eat and drink.

*Unacceptable Levels* filmmaker, Ed Brown, reveals that there are 80,000 chemicals on the market, and most of these have not been tested for their toxic effects on humans. Companies are free to put chemicals in consumer products without knowing whether they are safe or not. This is no small problem – this is a big issue that is greatly impacting the health of many, many individuals. [63]

Chemical consumer products are getting into our physiological systems in numerous ways. While we understand that high doses of chemicals can be lethal, the latest research reveals that even minute exposures can disrupt our normal genetic patterns and can create permanent changes in our hormonal systems. With up to 232 industrial chemicals floating around in our bodies, they can interfere with our reproductive systems, immune systems, childhood development, all of which can affect your physical, mental and emotional abilities. And do you know when people finally wake up and want to learn more about these? When their children experience learning disabilities or develop terminal threats. Should you really wait until this happens before being willing to do the research and do something about it? [64]

According to the Northwestern Health Sciences University:

- Cocamide DEA/Lauramide DEA, a foaming/cleansing agent found in baby wash, acne formulas, moisturizers, body scrubs, can create carcinogens
- Butylated hydroxytoluene, found in moisturizers, soaps, shaving creams, deodorants, skin care cleanser, and body wash, may cause eye and skin irritations
- Formaldehyde is found in antiperspirants, soaps, shaving creams, and shampoo and is considered a carcinogen that can damage DNA
- Parabens are found in many products and may cause skin irritations, impair fertility, and have been found in breast tumors
- Talc, a toxic chemical found in many powders, is a known carcinogen linked to ovarian cancer [65]

Don't be fooled into thinking that if it's expensive or the slick packaging says the product is "natural" it must be a safe product to use. Do the research and make sure the company has your health in mind with the creation of their product line. Go to www.ewg.org and let them help you determine the safety of your choice of products.

## What about sunscreens?

Sunscreen usage has risen dramatically for skin cancer prevention, according to EWG (Environmental Working Group, www.ewg.org), but cases have tripled from 7.89 in 1975 per 100,000 population to 23.57 in 2010.

With the many warnings of skin cancer, many of us look at the sun as our enemy. However, you need sunshine, and most people often do not get enough good daily sunshine. Exposure to the sun provides the body with Vitamin D3, which is necessary for building and maintaining strong and healthy bones. Vitamin D3 also plays an important role in the metabolism of calcium, as well as the functions of the heart, eyes and nervous system. Being outside in the early morning for fifteen to thirty minutes on a good brisk walk or bike is so good for adults and children too.

Overexposure by being in full sun between ten o'clock in the morning and four o'clock in the afternoon for extended periods of times without shade (when the sun's rays are the strongest) is not good for you or your skin. When the UV (ultraviolet) rays attack, free radicals can be created which are unstable oxygen molecules that have only one electron instead of two. Since electrons are found in pairs, these free radical molecules must raid other molecules for another electron. When the next molecule loses its electron to the first, it must also find another electron, and the process repeats itself. This process can damage and alter the functions of the cells, which can cause premature wrinkling and genetic cell damage as well.

However, are sunscreens the answer?

According to the research from EWG that published its 2014 guide in reviewing over 2000 sunscreens and 257 brands, 75 percent of these sunscreens contained toxic chemicals that put you at risk for many health issues. EWG stated that these readily absorb into the bloodstream and can create effects that include estrogen and hormone disruptors, skin irritations, allergic reactions, and damaging free radicals themselves. Many of them sold, as toxic as they are, can also be ineffective as a sunscreen. [66]

The following include some of the unsafe chemicals found in sunscreens:

- Oxybenzone
- Octinoxate (Octylmethoxycinnamate or Methoxycinnamate)
- Homosalate
- Octisalate
- Octocrylene [67]

If you have sunscreens with any of these ingredients, I strongly encourage you to discard them. Otherwise, use a good skin-protecting oil such as the Ultimate Skin Protection Oil in Chapter 32, which can provide nourishment and protection for your skin naturally.

Additionally, don't use sun blocks at all. Consider the fact that blocking the sun with high SPF can create a calcium deficiency due to the lack of vitamin D absorption.

Be smart:

- Get at least twenty minutes of full sunshine daily – go on a walk or run or bike ride
- Nourish your skin with the Ultimate Skin Protection Oil (see Chapter 32)

- Cover up with clothing if you are going to be out in the sun for extended periods of time.
- If you feel you need a sunscreen for those extended periods, choose a non-toxic sunscreen with a zinc or titanium base.
- If you do get burned, apply lavender essential oil (but only a pure therapeutic grade will provide the protection you need).

Would you like to know a really important secret about your body and the sun?

Let's start by addressing the functions of the liver. The liver is the largest organ in the human body (next to your skin), and its main functions are to help the body digest and use food, as well as purify the blood of wastes and poisons. Digested food travels from the small intestines to the liver. The liver stores some of the digested food from the blood and releases it back into the bloodstream when needed. The liver filters wastes and poisons from the blood, then must process it and dump it into the urinary track. When your liver becomes overloaded and full of toxins, it is released back into the body through the blood, and dumps it out into the fascia under your skin.

With a dirty, toxic, overloaded liver, which is caused by eating unhealthy and toxic foods and drinks, and using all kinds of chemical agents and skin products that are absorbed into the skin, the bloodstream ends up carrying these wastes throughout the body that settle in the skin. As your skin grabs the sunlight, it pulls up toxins to the surface, creating sunspots, or liver spots. We blame the sun for these ugly spots, whereas in reality, an unhealthy toxic liver is really to blame.

Instead of being grateful for the sun in working so hard to cleanse the toxicity from your liver and skin as it should naturally, simply because you have invited all these toxic substances into your body to begin with, most revert to treating the skin with yet more unhealthy chemicals and do everything to block and blame the sun, thus slathering on sunscreens that creates more toxic chemicals…and in the process adding even more to the toxic load of your body.

Your skin is a reflection of what is going on in the inside of your body. Sunscreens are NOT the answer to healthy skin – these won't ultimately prevent skin cancer. Studies show this. With healthier food choices, cleansing out the toxicity, eliminating toxic cleaners and body care, providing good tools of nourishment and essential oil compounds, you will have a healthier, vibrant skin. Respect the sun – you need it – it's good for you and will assist you if you allow it to. Listen to your body and treat it like you are truly a multi-million dollar machine because you are! Love yourself enough to protect your body and your environment.

About now, you might be saying "Okay you are telling me I ought to give up my comfort foods, my soft drinks, toss my synthetic supplements and medicines, and now you are going so far as telling me to discard my favorite body lotion and skin care too?"

Think about this. Does this give you a greater insight to why many children as well as adults are experiencing a variety of minor and major health issues? Can you see that there is a pattern of non-caring producers and manufactures that are interested in your money but could ultimately care less about your health?

A few years ago, I conducted a conference call series, and on the final call, I asked for comments from the attendees on what they had learned. One girl got all choked up and began with, "I'm angry!" I wasn't sure what she meant but we all waited patiently as she got her composure and continued to say how angry she felt when she went into the grocery store now realizing that our health is not considered when it came to foods, body care, and cleaners. It was just all about profit... it's true, and she knew it! You and I can be proactive and choose wisely because...

Every time you enter the grocery store – YOU VOTE! You vote on what foods this store should carry by the purchases you make!

Every time you go out to eat – YOU VOTE! You vote on the kind of foods and types of restaurants you want to stay in business!

Every time you get sick – YOU VOTE on healthcare! You vote through your purchases on what kind of medicines should be continued to be available: drugs, herbs, essential oils, etc.

Every time you make any type of purchase of any kind, a movie ticket, an article of clothing, etc. – YOU VOTE! Your choices, in your purchases, are messages sent to the producers and manufacturers to make more of what you are buying! Think about that!

I can tell you that I am very passionate about all of the choices we each make. If you want to see the world change for the better, it must start with you. Your vote is counted every time you shop, and your choices do determine what the manufactures are producing based on your purchases, so be choosy and choose to VOTE for health! Be open and invite others to make healthy choices as well.

What is a reliable solution for many of these areas?

Pure therapeutic-grade essential oils are antibacterial, anti-fungal, antimicrobial, antiviral, and anti-parasitic. If they are safe enough to ingest, they can make safer disinfecting and cleaning agents too for:

- air fresheners
- laundry detergents
- dish soaps
- cleansers
- carpet cleaners
- tile cleaners
- drain cleaners
- glass cleaners
- lotions
- sunscreens
- lip balms
- deodorants
- skin care
- and much more!

The fact that you can take pure therapeutic lemon essential oil into your body and cleanse your internal organs so effectively – but also use that same oil to clean your carpet as I shared earlier (better than anything else available), disinfect the counter tops, and more is just so amazing! What else can you do with lemon essential oil?

- Glass and mirror cleaner: put 2 drops lemon essential oil in an 8oz glass spritzer bottle with 1/2 cup white vinegar and 1/2 cup tap water – spray on glass, wipe with paper towels
- Gum resin remover: drop 1-2 drops lemon essential oil on jars that leave a gum resin after removing a label, rub and wash with warm water and soap
- Chewing gum: remove as much as possible first, then use a few drops lemon essential oil to loosen and remove the rest

Here's another simple tip I will share with you. It may blow you away as it does so many people I share this with. There is an awesome blend of essential oils that work so well in dispelling pathogens very effectively, which consists of clove, cinnamon, orange, rosemary, and eucalyptus. With 10 drops of this combination – or 2 drops of each of these individual oils – in an 8 oz. glass spritzer bottle filled with purified water, you can use this in multiple ways in your bathroom: disinfect the counter tops, the tile, the toilet, even disinfect the floors (several squirts with a wet water mop), use it as an air freshener, as a hand sanitizer, as well as a mouthwash! No joke! You've just replaced seven expensive, toxic products (or more) in your bathroom with 10 drops of essential oil in a bottle of water (cost is about $2, with the spritzer bottle $3). Same formula – safe enough for the toilet and your mouth too! Give it a try!

Here are some other suggestions with this same essential oil formula given above:

- Keep another bottle in your kitchen to use as a fruit and veggie wash (shake first before spritzing). Spritz on your produce and then wash it thoroughly to remove toxic residues and eliminate or lessen pathogens.

- Pour this formula in a 2 oz. spritzer bottle and keep it in your car. Although I don't recommend keeping your essential oils in your car because of possible heat damage, this is a small amount to keep in your console at all times and use effectively as a: hand sanitizer (after getting gas, before eating food), air freshener, or mouth spritz. Super effective, super inexpensive! Works so well! You have something that is safe, effective, inexpensive, and non-toxic too!

You can see that YOU HAVE A CHOICE in everything you do. You can choose nature and what it can produce for you instead of the toxic chemicals that are out there. This is reality, and YOU can do something about it if your body, as well as your children's bodies, are worth it! You can simply create many products, purchase non-toxic products, toss the harsh chemicals, and use common sense. You may live in a chemical world, but you can avoid many of the toxic effects by choosing nature.

## GOALS AND SUGGESTIONS

Do a complete home cleanse:

- Discard all chemical cleaners, soaps, and detergents that contain harmful components (most or all of them) and replace them with toxic-free alternatives, many of which you can make simply (see Chapter 31).
- Discard all pesticides, insecticides, etc. that pose a potential threat to your health and your family, and then replace them with simple solutions with nature.
- Discard all body care, skin care, hair care, oral care, nail care, etc., most of which are full of harmful chemicals that can pose serious threats to your health, then again replace them with safe, toxic-free skin products that do not contain these ingredients. For example recipes found in nature – see Chapter 32. If you need help, please visit: www.livingahealthylifestyle.com and we will assist you personally.

Removing toxic products from your home may be one of the most exhilarating things you can accomplish. You will ultimately feel like there has been a deep dark cloud lifted, you will feel more energy, you will feel your burdens lifted as you remove the toxic load and replenish your home with items that are toxic free. You will be much more effective in protecting your environment, your body, and those around you!

# UPLIFT

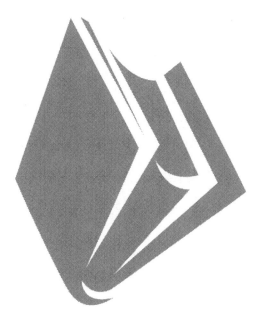

# Chapter 27

# YOUR MIND AND SOUL

I got this email from my dear friend Mary…

"I had lost all hope that I would be able to do the assignments required for my coaching certification course. Just reading a book in the last two years has been impossible for me. My concentration didn't last more than twenty minutes, so when I'd go back to pick up where I had stopped, my retention was scattered and meaningless. I had been given ninety days to fulfill this task. Here it was six weeks with only a 1/2 book read and no memory of it. Frustrated and confused, I lost all my confidence that I would be able to complete the assignments. I was once a successful Business Owner & Nurse!!

"You see, I'd had two strokes, with a concussion a few years ago. Now I was on my nutritional supplements, and was eating clean health foods, but still I had no focus. I wanted my former medications! This assignment overwhelmed me. I couldn't deal with it. I had stopped that 'crutch' 6 months ago, and I was not about to start back up on the meds again. I told Erleen I couldn't do it, at least not on a time schedule. I felt relief, but sad that I was basically giving up.

"Then, I received a notice from Erleen that she wanted the assignments finished in September so she could announce those who had completed the certification at convention. I WANTED my NAME announced just to avoid the embarrassment of my team knowing I failed! I prayed that night. The next morning, it came to me!

"I had frankincense essential oil and an oil blend specific to my cellular needs. I had read these were effective in passing the blood brain barrier. I decided to alternate each of the oils, applying sublingual and to the roof of my mouth several times each day.

"I only had twelve days now to complete the assignment. I told myself to be Optimistic. I found that each day the data was coming back to me. I was able to complete the assignment in just ten days from start to finish, two days before the new deadline.

"Where ninety days seemed impossible, ten days became achievable for me. Thanks to these amazing essential oils for assisting my brain! Thank you Erleen for pushing my 'motivation button'."

Mary brings out many important factors that were foundational for her success:

- she prayed
- she had read and studied previously, so the answers came easily
- she reached for essential oils as a well-documented support she trusted
- she was optimistic and believed she could do what she needed to do
- she moved forward with determination

And because of this, Mary triumphed and achieved her goal!

## PRAYER AND MEDITATION

If you want to accomplish more in this life and travel on a more certain path, then consider spending some quiet time daily to communicate spirit to spirit with your God, and Creator. If you desire help ongoing, then prayer and meditation are not only important daily but throughout your day. To accomplish this best, go to a place where:

- you can be alone
- you can think without distractions
- you can be comfortable

Picture your Creator in your mind and speak to him as a literal person who is listening to you. Tell him what you are feeling from your heart, and have a heartfelt conversation with him. Thank him, confide in him, express your gratitude and love to him. Listen for answers – they will come quietly through thoughts and impressions in your mind.

After many days and hours of debate while our Founding Fathers were working to compose a Constitution for America, Benjamin Franklin made this statement to George Washington, the leader of the Constitutional Convention: "I have lived, Sir, a long time and the longer I live, the more convincing proofs I see of this truth – that God governs in the affairs of men. And if a sparrow cannot fall to the ground without his notice, is it probable that an empire can rise without his aid?"

How about you? Can you really fulfill your mission alone, or do you need divine help?

Through prayer and meditation, you can:

- find out God's will for you in fulfilling your mission in life
- find forgiveness for your mistakes and shortcomings
- find strength in fulfilling your tasks
- find direction in pathways never thought of previously
- find purpose in your pursuits
- find peace as you meet challenges
- find personal answers to questions you have

Taking time daily to pray and meditate can provide a daily "spiritual cleanse" and help you know more clearly what your heart is made of, what is truly important to you, what defines you, and where your strength truly lies. And as you experience this on a daily basis, you will be more capable of feeling more love, patience, understanding, and empathy for individuals. You will be able to communicate better because you have been able to communicate spiritually. You will be able to mentor better when you have been mentored. You will be able to be more understanding since you have been understood. You will be able to forgive others more willingly because you have been forgiven. That is the power of prayer.

## READ AND STUDY

What makes most of us want to be better and to commit to making changes? It usually always comes through someone else who has traveled a road or done a task that inspires us. This is the power of reading good books!

Those who want to make a difference in their own lives and make an impact on the world are readers. They learn from the great philosophers, scientists, leaders of their day, and people who have overcome extraordinary challenges. It's an attribute of successful people to be uplifted and inspired, then, in turn, uplift and inspire others.

The world needs more leaders who are willing to develop new habits, improve skills, who are much more drawn to reading a book of self-development than doing other time wasting activities. A leader is one who will "Learn it, Live it, and Lift others", is willing to lead out on new pathways, discover new territories, passionate about doing good for mankind, and making a difference in the world.

Here are some great books I highly recommend for your reading as a start:

- *Traditional Foods are Your Best Medicine*, Ronald R. Schmid, N.D.
- *Food and Behavior*, Barbara Reed Stitt
- *Modern Essentials*, Aroma Tools
- *Emotions and Essential Oils*, Enlighten
- *The Slight Edge*, Jeff Olsen
- *How to Win Friends and Influence People*, Dale Carnegie
- *The Greatest Salesman in the World*, Og Mandino

Get into the habit of reading eight to ten pages or more of a good book every day. Set aside a time, make that appointment with yourself as your education hour. Learn from good books, webinars, and research. And if this book inspires you to share this information with others in a leadership and business aspect, then consider these three areas of education:

- Learn all about wellness products, essential oils, and different wellness modalities.
- Learn all about your business and how to be effective in your communication skills.
- Learn self-development and leadership skills and how to become an effective leader.

When it comes to research and information, there is so much available today that sometimes it can be daunting – but that's also when learning becomes fun. Take the time to research some of the information you have been learning throughout this book. Note the intents and motives of information that you read and research – does it inspire you and cause you to take action? Does it resonate? Is it truth?

LEARN it, LIVE it, and LIFT others – this is a key for true success!

## ESSENTIAL OILS AND HOW THEY CAN AFFECT YOUR EMOTIONS

Aroma therapy is a powerful tool that has been found to be effective for the brain, emotions and many body responses for thousands of years. Smell can actually influence emotions, mood, and memory faster and more effectively than anything else. Scents can take you back to your childhood and bring up memories good or bad: the smell of fresh baked cinnamon rolls may remind you of Christmas at Grandma's house, or the smell of a new bookstore might remind you of your first day of school. Smells influence emotions, your mood, and your brain.

As you inhale the aroma of an essential oil, the molecules travel up your nose, stimulating the nerves of the olfactory membranes which then trigger electrical impulses to the olfactory bulb in the brain. Those impulses are transmitted to the amygdala – where emotions and memory are stored – and to other parts of the limbic system.

Since your brain's limbic system also controls your blood pressure, heart rate, breathing, stress levels, and hormone balance, essential oils can have profound effects physiologically and psychologically. Odors stimulate the release of hormones and neuro-chemicals that can greatly impact mood and behavior. [68]

Quality essential oils of pure therapeutic grade will offer you the best results. As mentioned previously, many synthetic oils can actually cause negative reactions and effects.

You can find great therapeutic benefits aromatically simply by opening a bottle of essential oil and smelling it, placing a drop in your hand and inhaling, placing a few drops in a diffuser with water, as well as applying essential oils topically on your wrist, back of neck, and/or behind your ear lobes. Here are just a few examples of possible benefits especially for the brain, mood, and emotions:

- <u>Basil</u>: calming for anxious and overwhelmed, supportive for the drained and exhausted
- <u>Bergamot</u>: ignites optimism and confidence, uplifting and encouraging
- <u>Black Pepper</u>: excellent for suppressing addictions, physical or mental
- <u>Cedarwood</u>: grounding and strengthening, promoting unity
- <u>Clary Sage</u>: dispelling confusion and discouragement, opening new ideas and creativity
- <u>Eucalyptus</u>: opens and supports the respiratory channels
- <u>Frankincense</u>: opens the memory for understanding, wisdom and knowledge, provides feelings of love and protection, enhances prayer and meditation, opens spiritual channels
- <u>Geranium</u>: facilitates trust in relationships, encourages love, connection and forgiveness
- <u>Grapefruit</u>: curbs emotional eating, promotes integrity and taking responsibility
- <u>Helichrysum</u>: provides emotional and spiritual healing and transformation
- <u>Lavender</u>: calms insecurities and fears, releasing tension, liberating self-inflicted imprisonment
- <u>Lemon</u>: dispels confusion, supports mental focus and clarity, elevating
- <u>Lemongrass</u>: supports cleansing physically, emotionally and spiritually
- <u>Melissa</u>: awakening to the soul of your purpose and mission for life
- <u>Patchouli</u>: grounding, stabilizing, calming fears and nervous tension
- <u>Peppermint</u>: invigorating, uplifting, and relieving of pain emotionally and physically
- <u>Roman Chamomile</u>: centering, empowering, calming, soul supporting

- <u>Rose</u>: promotes love, charity, warmth, compassion, meditation
- <u>Sandalwood:</u> stress reducing, calming to the mind, prepares the spirit for communion with Deity
- <u>Tangerine</u>: encourages creativity and spontaneity, uplifting mood
- <u>Thyme</u>: powerful emotional cleanser of hate, anger, resentment, negativity
- <u>Vetiver</u>: grounding while emotional liberating, providing focus
- <u>White Fir</u>: unearthing of negative inherited patterns, providing spiritual support
- <u>Wild Orange</u>: inspires and elevates the mood while reducing stress
- <u>Ylang Ylang</u>: powerful for releasing strong emotions from the past, nurturing feelings of love.[69]

Overall, just a drop or two of pure therapeutic-grade essential oils can enhance your learning, increase your endurance, support your emotions, and provide mental, emotional and physical strengthening. Try them and see for yourself.

## BE OPTIMISTIC

Henry Ford was a huge believer in positive thinking and how it is paramount in accomplishing anything we do. He said: "If you think you can or you think you can't, you're right. It's the thinking that makes it so." This is true in every facet of your life: family and marriage, weight loss, business success, and more!

Here is the most amazing secret: The most successful people in history ALL have one thing in common – they believe they can succeed, they believe in themselves, they envision success, and they KNOW they will get there!

Unsuccessful people, on the other hand, blame their parents, the economy, their childhood, the bank, politics, on and on. Yet you create your world through your thoughts...mentally before physically. This is not voodoo, and it's not new age stuff. The physical outcome of your day is mentally created by you personally first.

What you think about and believe is what you create in your life even if you don't know it. Your unconscious brain does not know the difference between your past experiences or your future experiences, but YOUR BRAIN DOES MANIFEST WHAT YOU THINK ABOUT ALL THE TIME. So if you constantly remember your fears, your frustrations, your anger due to a situation, your failings – you continue to breed fear, frustration, anger, self-doubt, etc. Instead, if you consciously envision your desires, focus on your goals in the present as if you are already there, live them now, be there now, then your mind attracts and creates this vision, it becomes real – it manifests itself! This, in essence, is the true meaning of faith – doubting nothing, fully believing in the manifestation of your goal. And the beauty of this is that if your thoughts and your belief really do create your physical outcome, you have much more control over your destiny.

Kevin Trudeau teaches in "Your Wish is Your Command" CD series that the brain is a transmitter and receiver of vibrational frequencies. Everything on earth is made of energy and frequencies, and every cell in the body emits different frequencies. Your brain puts out a frequency picked up by other brains instantaneously, faster than the speed of light. We often call this the LAW OF ATTRACTION: whatever frequency you emit, the exact frequency is drawn back to you magnetically. Because of this, "you get what you think about most of the time," and "you become what you think about most of the time." But this clearly depends on your:

- Increased power and intensity – thinking about it all the time
- Increasing your duration long enough to activate – constantly transmitting a frequency
- Having complete faith and vision of your success without any ounce of doubt.[70]

If you activate your goals and vision with intensity and duration, you will achieve them – there's no way not to if you:

- Have a burning desire – really want something bad enough
- Feel good about what you are creating, that it's for the right reason and purpose

- Match your self-talk with your goals/desires/belief (you can't envision success but be thinking you will fail)
- Have 100% Belief that you will receive – You will get there if you believe you will!

"Ask, and it shall be given you; seek, and ye shall find; knock, and it shall be opened unto you" Matthew 7:7

"For whatsoever a man soweth, that shall he also reap." Galatians 6:7

"If any of you lack wisdom, let him ask of God, that giveth to all men liberally, and upbraideth not; and it shall be given him. But let him ask in faith, nothing wavering. For he that wavereth is like a wave of the sea driven with the wind and tossed." James 1:5-6 [71]

"If you want things in your life to change, you're going to have to change things in your life." [72] You can't keep doing the same things every day and expect different results.

JD Houston said, "If you want something in your life you've never had, you have to do something you have never done".

Being successful is a decision. Richard Brooke, said in *Mach II With Your Hair on Fire,* "Everything changed for me when I developed the willingness to train myself to think like a successful person." THINK SUCCESS!

- Begin your day: Focus on what you desire – think about it all the time
- Use positive words, speak positively all the time
- Read good books daily, listen to good CDs daily, eat wholesome foods, exercise and do positive activities that will create positive energy physically, emotionally and mentally
- Associate with people who talk positively, who will support your efforts
- Watch your feelings...... YOU MUST FEEL GOOD about the goals you want to achieve!
- Begin and end each day with prayer, meditation and gratitude – and be grateful for everything, even your challenges.

You are meant to be a creator each and every day – you are always creating. The question is what? What outcomes are you creating today with your thoughts? Make your thoughts count!

"What outcomes are you creating with your thoughts? Make your thoughts count!"

## BE DETERMINED TO SUCCEED

I love what my sweet friend Annie sent me:

"'In order to succeed, your desire for success should be greater than your fear of failure.' (Bill Crosby). I love this quote and think it rings true for all of us. It doesn't matter what you do, where you are going or how you wanna get there, if you don't believe that you can succeed, it's inevitable, you're gonna fail!

"When I started building my business four months ago, I set goals for myself, and I wrote them down. I look at them all the time, and my leaders hold me accountable for them. That for me is huge. You have to have a plan and a way to get there. Don't sell yourself short, do the work, and you will see the results. It may be at the last hour that everything comes to fruition, but if you've put forth the effort and plan to succeed, you will!!!!

"I am not doing anything special, just working hard, holding lots of classes (one which NOBODY, yes nobody showed up to) and I contact A LOT of people. For any success, you have to put yourself out there and let people know why you are so passionate about what you are doing. Don't ever quit on a bad day! We all have them, but remember that it too shall pass.

"Just keep doing the little things, one step at a time, set you goals high and be accountable for them! Be the best YOU, you can be!"

Life is a journey, not a destination. However, this journey has many destinations along the way. Goals are important as a way to progress and arrive at new horizons in life's journey. Planning and achieving your goals with determination can be just as easy as planning a successful vacation to Alaska.

You usually create the entire event before you get there – this doesn't mean every step, or that you experience every detail – that is the gift that comes along the way. But you mentally create the whole experience and make the physical preparations to make it happen BEFORE you ever get there:

- planning travel flights, transportation
- shopping beforehand
- arranging sitting plans for the children, pets, the home
- scheduling time off from work, contacting workers, working around events
- packing clothes for the duration according to your activities
- having a day-to-day plan of activities: sites, hotels, reservations
- having checkpoints along the way: to the airport, to the first layover, second layover, etc.
- pre-planning connections with persons or contacts while there
- making plans for the day of your return, whomever will pick you up and so forth

Most likely, it will happen just as you have planned, even though there are always adjustments in details along the way. But you create this whole scenario mentally before physically, and it will go pretty much as you have created it. If you instead, just let it happen, then that's how it will go as well. Without any plans, things may go well or they may not – you won't be either happy or disappointed because you have no goal nor any expectations.

Now take time to put the same kind of work and detail into setting your goals. If you have a list of checkpoints along the way that you cross off, you will for sure see the progress and find success.

Thomas Jefferson, Benjamin Franklin, George Washington and many men of their day lived by their own creeds, habits, and words of wisdom that they self-created.

At the age of 20, Benjamin Franklin created a system to develop his character which governed his entire life. He called them his thirteen virtues:

1. Temperance. Eat not to dullness; drink not to elevation.
2. Silence. Speak not but what may benefit others or yourself; avoid trifling conversation.

3.  Order. Let all your things have their places; let each part of your business have its time.
4.  Resolution. Resolve to perform what you ought; perform without fail what you resolve.
5.  Frugality. Make no expense but to do good to others or yourself; i.e., waste nothing.
6.  Industry. Lose no time; be always employed in something useful; cut off all unnecessary actions.
7.  Sincerity. Use no hurtful deceit; think innocently and justly, and, if you speak, speak accordingly.
8.  Justice. Wrong none by doing injuries, or omitting the benefits that are your duty.
9.  Moderation. Avoid extremes; forbear resenting injuries so much as you think they deserve.
10. Cleanliness. Tolerate no uncleanliness in body, clothes, or habitation.
11. Tranquility. Be not disturbed at trifles, or at accidents common or unavoidable.
12. Chastity. Rarely use venery but for health or offspring, never to dullness, weakness, or the injury of your own or another's peace or reputation.
13. Humility. Imitate Jesus and Socrates.

What about you?

Are you mentally creating positive outcomes in your life, or is life just happening to you?

What are the virtues and traits that are important to you?

What are you doing to uplift and strengthen your body, mind and soul on a daily basis?

# GOALS AND SUGGESTIONS

Look at the areas discussed in this chapter. What do you need to do in each of these areas to uplift your mind and help you reach your goals?

- prayer and meditation
- reading daily and better educating yourself
- using essential oils for emotional, mental, and physical support
- being optimistic and believing in yourself
- being determined to succeed in reaching your goals
- Create a plan of action. If you feel you need a mentor to guide you through the process, visit: www.livingahealthylifestyle.com

Create a mission statement or your own rules to live by which may include:

- important character traits that you want to maintain or develop
- your values, roles and responsibilities
- your goals, dreams, life's mission

Write out you mission statement, fine tune it and post it somewhere so you can read it often to act as a guide for your life.

# CONCLUSION

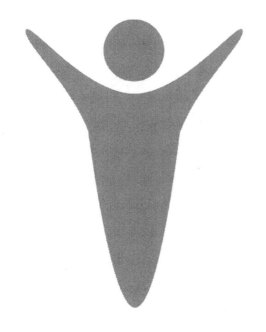

# Chapter 28

# YOUR BODY IS A SYSTEM

Your body is a SYSTEM, and as mentioned earlier, just like a car, all of the components are important. They all work together synergistically! You can live without an ear, your eyes, one kidney – yes, and many do! But it's not as easy as when all body functions are in place in proper working order.

Here's one last very important thing for you to understand.

"Human Beings have an Autonomic Nervous System (ANS) that is actually comprised of three separate subsystems, the Parasympathetic Nervous System (PNS), the Sympathetic Nervous System (SNS) and the Enteric Nervous System (ENS)." [73]

The PNS is responsible for your body's activities concerning "rest and digest". In a normal happy state, the digestive system runs smoothly, you can relax and sleep well.

The SNS is responsible for stimulating your body's "fight or flight" response. In a normal happy state, it will give your body the energy it needs and provide balance with these other systems, which we call homeostasis.

The ENS has been described as your 'second brain,' which communicates with the central nervous system (CNS) through the parasympathetic – by way of the vagus nerve.

The Enteric Nervous System consists of sheaths of neurons embedded in the walls of your gut – or alimentary canal – which goes from your esophagus to your anus. Along with the chemical processes that are a part of the digestive system such as breaking down food, extracting nutrients, removing wastes, you have over 100 million neurons in your gut – which is more than in the Central Nervous System itself. These enable you to have feelings and sensations often overlooked as coming from your gut. [74]

In other words, your digestive system does much more than digest your foods – it plays a key role in your emotional and mental health as well as diseases and dysfunctions experienced throughout your body.

Your gut and brain are in constant communication with each other. The Enteric Nervous System uses thirty or more neurotransmitters just like your brain, and a big part of your emotions are influenced by what goes on in your gut. For example, 95 percent of your body's serotonin – a neurotransmitter responsible for mood, emotions, sleep, and more – is found in your gut.

About 90 percent of the signals that pass along the vagus nerve come from your gut to your brain, not from your brain to your gut and that's why many times you feel butterflies or real nervous signals from your gut – your "second brain" – that act as a guide for many of the decisions you make in your life. [75]

While it's not certain which comes first – poor gut health or poor mental health – we do know that your nervous system and digestive system are connected. This means what you put into your digestive tract – what you eat and drink – greatly influences your brain-gut communication, your behavior, your energy, your mood, your emotions, your health, your entire system. They work together and are greatly affected by your lifestyle choices!

Your BODY SYSTEM is your life gift! It works optimally or minimally according to how you:

- NOURISH: what kind of foods you choose to eat
- CLEANSE: how efficient your body removes toxicity
- BUILD: the balance of nutrients you provide
- SUPPORT: the kind of care you use for target support
- STRENGTHEN: the amount of physical exercise you do daily
- PROTECT: keeping your body safe from external toxic substances
- UPLIFT: how you think and support your brain

I like to think of my different cells as little internal elves, working happily along within me in all my different bodily processes that take place. Everything is cellular......everything is chemistry. Cells, organs, systems work happily or they struggle with overload.

182

After you read the following question, close your eyes for a full minute and visualize:

<u>Based on how you are doing in each of these seven areas, how do you think your cells (little elves) are working in each of your systems in your body?</u>

- Are they working happily?
- Are they stressed and overloaded?
- Are you ready to make some changes?
- Have you really learned the secrets of healthy, happy people?
- Are you ready to live a healthy, happy lifestyle yourself?
- Are you ready to be the change you want to see in the world?

If you are ready…let's get started!

1) You must have a HUGE DESIRE big enough to make the changes no matter what!
2) You must TRAIN YOUR MIND TO THINK DIFFERENTLY! This will be much easier than you think if you are teachable, and you have a huge desire.
3) You will need to BE CHOOSY even though others may not be. However, this all depends on your attitude and if you have the nerve to say "come learn with me", or "I'd love to have your support".
4) Continue to EDUCATE YOURSELF because this will give you the reasons to make good decisions.
5) You must have a PERSONAL MENTOR to guide you through the process. It's a rare occasion that you might succeed on your own – you will need a mentor!

Don't procrastinate. Tell me you are ready to live the Healthy Happy Life right here:

<u>www.livingahealthylifestyle.com</u>

# LET'S GET STARTED

# Chapter 29

# WHERE TO BEGIN

Now that we have the foundation, let's get started – here's how!

1. Do a home cleanse (junk foods, frozen foods, chemical cleansers, chemical body products......pretend you are moving, clean it all out) – most of your success will come from having done this...remove the toxins and temptations all at once. You are starting your journey to wellness, and toxic foods and products are not allowed to take space in your home or your body. Take this seriously. If you don't like the box you are in, then you have to step out of it. Divorce those items that are not in your best interest, marry those that love your cells and body! (And don't give them to your neighbors – you want them to join you right?)

2. Ask others to support your lifestyle change. Let people know up front that you are excited to be making some positive changes, ask them to come along, let them know you are still learning and you'd like a workout partner.

3. Find a new place to shop. This again will make a HUGE difference in your success. Be serious, find a good healthy store that has an organic, whole food focus. Shop at the organic produce section for most of your food items...or grow an organic garden. You may initially spend more but you will SAVE more in the long run for sure! See the Dirty Dozen Pesticide Foods to Avoid list in Chapter 25.

4. Shop whole. You don't need a whole book of recipes to get you started. You just need to think WHOLE: whole fruits and vegetables, whole beans, whole grains, whole chunks of meat, whole

nuts and seeds, oil, vinegar, salt, etc. When you do this, you become a gourmet cook, believe it or not...but it's super simple!

5. The most dynamic and secret ingredients of these recipes are essential oils... only those with the highest therapeutic quality, safe for internal use. These will support and accelerate better digestion, cleansing, fortifying your bodily functions plus provide great flavor! Get them so you can enjoy the benefits.

6. Prepare ahead of time...don't make this a problem. Most people fail here because they have relied on so-called convenience foods as the norm, not the emergency. Think ahead, plan ahead, carry fresh fruit, raw nuts, etc. with you so you are not tempted to break down at your starving point for inferior foods.

7. Events, parties, dinners, social setting all have food. Here's what you can do: first, choose the best of what's available, and if there's nothing good, "no thanks" with a smile is a good response! If there's an opportunity, offer to bring something healthy. If that's not an option, you can often find out ahead of time what the menu is and plan accordingly. The more you bring the healthy stuff, you will be surprised that people will admire you for leading the way. If not, forgive them for not understanding your big why.

8. We travel the world and people will ask what you eat that's healthy...guess what? There are whole foods ALL around the world, if you are looking for them, and they are in almost every quality store and restaurant so just look for them. Focus on the good stuff and forget the rest.

## CLEANSING DIET: CREATING MEAL PLANS

This is a menu guide for healthy eating, cleansing your body, as well as putting your body into fat burning mode.

1. Make sure you get a small amount of good clean protein with each meal or snack
2. Vary your protein throughout the day (example choices: 1 meat, 1 eggs, 1 beans, 1-2 small portions of raw nuts, 1-2 portions of sprouts, etc.)

3. Make sure your carbs are complex carbs – whole grains, vegetables, fruits, beans (no refined sugar or flour, whole-grain breads only on a rare occasion)
4. Concentrate on lots of vegetables (especially greens and more greens), some fruits, baked or steamed vegetables, then protein as the condiment.

## Breakfasts Ideas

- Smoothies: fresh vegetable and fruit (see Sunrise Smoothie recipe)
- Raw fruits with raw almond butter as a dip (or soaked almonds)
- Omelets with fresh vegetables (kale, zucchini, spinach, red pepper, etc.)
- Wraps (lettuce wraps filled with scrambled egg, hummus, vegetable strips, hot sauce)

## Snack

- If you've had fruit for breakfast: celery or carrot sticks with a few raw/soaked almonds
- If you've had vegetables for breakfast: apples or other with a few raw/soaked almonds

## Lunch – fresh greens and clean protein will keep cravings under control

- Green Salads – top with baked chicken, or drained beans, sprouts and seeds or nuts – salad bar style!
- Green salad topped with raw sunflower/pumpkin seeds, and baked sweet potato
- Wraps (like breakfast)
- Salmon salad – green salad with 2-3 additional vegetables and previous baked salmon

## Snack

- Large organic apple or pear,
- 1-2 squares Energy Bars,
- Healthy Fudge, Protein Bites (only 1-inch squares), or

- Cinnamon Trio (golf ball chunk)
- Leftover Sunrise Smoothie

## Dinner – small to medium amount of protein, the less combinations the better

- Any of the lunch menu suggestions
- Baked chicken or fish, large green salad, steamed broccoli or squash, etc.
- Soup (full of vegetables, maybe some brown rice or quinoa, chicken), lots of fresh vegetables
- Small bowl of beans, large green salad with fresh celery (good for digestion)

## Think you need dessert?

- Try 8-10 raw almonds
- Herbal tea (peppermint or toothpick amount of peppermint essential oil), stevia
- A 1-inch square Energy Bar, Healthy Fudge, Protein Bites
- On a rare occasion, go for the Coconut Ice Delicious – this is good for you, but not at ten o'clock at night!

# Chapter 30

# SUPER FOODS FOR HEALTHY HAPPY PEOPLE

**SUNRISE SMOOTHIE**

A Great Way to Start Your Day

- 3 cups water
- 1/2 cup raw, soaked almonds (soaked improves digestibility, but raw is okay too)
- Handful of baby greens or spinach leaves
- 1 heaping scoop good quality protein powder
- 1 small scoop dry greens powder
- 1 large carrot, cut into chunks
- 1 large stalk celery, cut into chunks
- 1 large apple, cut into chunks
- 4-5 pitted dates or 1/2 dropper stevia
- 1/2 banana, peeled, fresh or frozen (optional)
- 8 drops grapefruit, wild orange, lemon or tangerine essential oil
- 2 teaspoon omega-3 oil (optional)
- 2-3 cups frozen fruit blend (berries, papaya, mango, pineapple, peaches, etc)

Place ingredients in blender, except frozen fruit. Blend on high until smooth, add frozen fruit and blend well again. If the recipe makes too much for one meal, refrigerate and enjoy for your mid-afternoon snack. A Sunrise Smoothie will grow on you. If it's not your favorite breakfast now, believe me, it won't take long until it is! This is so delicious, so filling, and is the means to fueling your day with full energy!

## ENERGY BARS

Everyone loves these – great mid-afternoon snack with half an apple!

- 1 1/2 cups honey
- 2 cups raw almond butter or other nut butter
- 8-10 drops wild orange, cinnamon or lemon essential oil
- 2 drops ginger essential oil
- 1 cup good quality protein powder
- 4 cups rolled oats

If honey is hardened, lightly warm in saucepan just to soften, but not get HOT. Stir in nut butter until smooth, then add essential oil and mix until smooth again. Stir in protein powder and oats. Mix thoroughly and spread in a 8" x 12" glass dish. Chill well; cut into 1-inch squares as a serving.

## HEALTHY FUDGE

Very satisfying chunk of nutrition!

- 1 cup raw almond butter
- 1/2 cup tahini (sesame butter)
- 4 drops cinnamon essential oil
- 4 drops bergamot essential oil
- 2 tablespoons black strap molasses
- 2 tablespoon honey or pure maple syrup
- 2 tablespoons mixed greens powder
- 2 tablespoons sunflower seeds or hemp seeds
- 2 tablespoons sesame seeds
- 2 tablespoons pumpkin seeds
- 1 tablespoon chia seeds
- optional: 1 teaspoon of bee pollen and/or ginseng granules
- 1/3 cup good quality protein powder

In medium-large mixing bowl, combine first 6 ingredients Fold in remaining ingredients and mix well Press in a 8 x 8 inch glass dish. Chill and cut into 1 inch squares as a serving.

## PROTEIN BITES

Nice little yummy treat!

- 1 cup almond butter
- 1/2 cup raw honey
- 3 drops wild orange essential oil
- 1/4 teaspoon salt
- 1/2 cup finely shredded coconut
- 1/4 cup raw sunflower seeds or hemp seeds
- 1/4 cup dried currants or raisins
- 2 tablespoons chia seeds

Finely shredded coconut or sesame seeds. **In medium mixing bowl, combine all ingredients except last. Stir until well mixed. Roll into balls and coat with the coconut or sesame seeds. Store in the refrigerator and enjoy when a small bit of protein is needed.**

## CINNAMON TRIO

This is a great grab-n-go, instead of packaged bars!

- 1 cup each of 3 raw nuts (cashews, almonds, pecans, walnuts, pistachios, etc.)
- 1 cup each of 3 raw seeds (sunflower, sesame, pumpkin)
- 1 cup each of 3 dried fruits (raisins, golden raisins, dry cranberries, currents, mango)
- 1 1/2 cup honey
- 1/4 teaspoon salt
- 2 Tablespoons butter or non-hydrogenated spread
- 1 teaspoon vanilla
- 4 drops cinnamon essential oil (must be meant for internal use)

Combine all 9 cups of nuts, seeds and fruits in a large bowl. In large saucepan, combine honey, salt, butter, and vanilla; bring to boil and boil to soft ball stage (when the color starts to change from golden to light brown). Remove from heat and stir in cinnamon oil. Drizzle over nut mix and stir to combine well. Serve on a plate pulled apart or keep this made up in a covered glass dish on the counter, and when someone needs a quick snack to go – it's ready!

## HUMMUS

Awesome dip for veggies and whole grain/seed crackers!

- 2 cups canned or cooked chickpeas, well drained
- 3 Tablespoons sesame seeds or tahini (raw sesame butter)
- 2 cloves garlic
- 3/4 teaspoon salt
- 1 teaspoon red pepper sauce or pinch cayenne pepper
- 1 Tablespoon olive oil
- ¾ cup water
- 5-6 drops lemon essential oil
- 5-6 drop lime essential oil

Blend all ingredients in blender until smooth, adding additional water, if needed. Spoon into a jar or a dish; and is best if chilled well first. Serve as a dip with freshly cut vegetables: carrots, celery, cucumbers, red pepper, broccoli, etc.

### Hummus Variations

- Jalapeno-Cilantro Hummus – Add 1 tsp. cumin, handful cilantro, and ¼ fresh jalapeño to blender
- Chipotle Hummus – Omit red pepper sauce; add 1 small Chipotle Pepper in Adobo Sauce & blend

## FRESH MEXICAN SALSA

This is a perfect tasting salsa!

- 10-12 plum tomatoes, finely diced
- 4 green onions, sliced
- 3 cloves garlic, minced

- Small handful cilantro, chopped fine
- 3 jalapenos, tops removed, chopped fine
- 3-4 drops lime essential oil
- 1 drop cilantro essential oil
- Toothpick black pepper essential oil
- ¾ -1 teaspoon salt (to taste)

With food processor or by hand, prepare first 5 ingredients and place in bowl. Add seasonings to taste. Chill well or serve at once with organic corn chips, brown rice chips, or hearty seed crackers.

## SPICY GUACAMOLE

Tasty as a dip or topping!

- 6 large diced avocados, mashed
- 4 plum tomatoes, diced
- 1/4 cup fine chopped red onion
- 1/2 cup fine chopped red bell pepper
- 1/4 cup fine chopped cilantro
- 1 small can sliced black olives
- 1/2 teaspoon garlic powder
- 1/4 teaspoon salt
- 3 drops lime essential oil
- Toothpick black pepper essential oil
- 1 teaspoon hot red pepper sauce

In medium bowl, mash avocados until creamy. Add all other ingredients and mix well. Chill if time allows before serving.

## MEXICAN SALAD

Great make-and-take salad for a crowd!

- 1 cup cooked black beans, drained, rinsed and drained well
- 2 Tablespoons olive oil
- 2 cloves garlic, minced or pressed

- 4-5 drops lime essential oil
- 1 drop black pepper essential oil
- 1 drop cilantro or coriander essential oil
- 1 teaspoon salt
- 2-3 teaspoons hot red pepper sauce (depending on hotness desired)
- 1/2 cup cooked non-GMO corn, drained
- 1 large red bell pepper, diced
- 1 large avocado, diced
- 1/2 cup chopped cilantro
- 4 green onions, sliced with tops
- 1 can sliced black olives
- 4-5 cups finely torn green leaf lettuce

In large salad bowl, combine first 8 ingredients. Layer the remaining ingredients without stirring. Just before serving, toss all together.

## CHINESE SALAD

Another great make-and-take salad for a crowd!

- 2 Tablespoon soy sauce or Braggs liquid aminos
- 2 Tablespoon olive oil
- 4 drops lemon essential oil
- 1 drop ginger essential oil
- 1/2 teaspoon garlic powder
- 1/4 teaspoon salt
- 1 cup cooked and chilled brown rice
- 1 cup sliced black olives
- 1 cup snow peas
- 1 cup broccoli florets
- 1/2 cup chopped red pepper
- 1/2 cup sliced raw almonds or cashew pieces
- 3 green onions, chopped
- 3 cup chopped green leaf lettuce

In salad bowl, toss combine first 6 ingredients. Layer on the cooked rice, and then add the vegetables. Toss just before serving.

## GREEK SALAD

Yum – great Greek flavor!

- 2 Tablespoons olive oil
- 6 drops lemon essential oil
- 1 drop rosemary essential oil
- 1 teaspoon salt
- 1/2 cup fresh snipped basil
- 1/4 teaspoon coarse ground black pepper
- 8 oz. organic tofu, drained and cubed
- 1/2 bunch green leaf lettuce, torn
- 1 cucumber, diced
- 2 plum tomatoes, diced
- 1/4 purple onion, diced
- 1 can black or Greek olives, whole or halved, and drained

In small bowl, combine oils, salt, basil, and pepper; add tofu and toss. In salad bowl, place other prepared ingredients.Just before serving, pour on oils and tofu mixture, and then gently toss and serve.

## HERBAL VINAIGRETTE DRESSING

- 1/2 cup cold pressed mild flavor olive oil
- 1/4 cup water
- 1/4 cup apple cider vinegar or balsamic vinegar
- 6 drops lemon or wild orange essential oil
- 1 drop rosemary or coriander essential oil
- 1 Tablespoon honey (slightly rounded)
- 3/4-1 teaspoon salt

Combine all ingredients in a jar and shake well before serving.

## CREAMY ITALIAN DRESSING

- 1/2 cup cold pressed mild flavor olive oil
- 1/4 cup water
- 1/4 cup apple cider vinegar or balsamic vinegar
- 6 drops lemon essential oil
- 1 Tablespoon honey (slightly rounded)
- 2 teaspoon liquid lecithin
- 3/4-1 teaspoon salt
- 1 teaspoon dry bell pepper flakes (in spice department: Sweet pepper flakes)

Place all ingredients in blender bowl, blend well, and chill.

## PLAIN KALE CHIPS

These are yummy and expensive, but simple to make, and what a savings!

- 1 large bunch kale, washed well, torn from stem
- 2 Tablespoons olive oil
- 3 drops lemon or lime essential oil
- Salt & Pepper

Prepare dehydrator at 115 degrees F, or preheat oven to 200 degrees F. Wash kale and pat dry with paper towels; place in large bowl. Mix oils and seasonings together. Drizzle on and massage in kale. Dehydrate until crisp or bake 45-50 minutes

## CHEESY KALE CHIPS

- 1 large bunch kale, washed well, torn from stem
- 3/4 cup water
- 1 cup raw cashews
- 1 teaspoon salt
- 1 teaspoon Braggs liquid aminos
- 1 teaspoon onion powder
- 1/2 teaspoon cumin powder
- 3 drops lemon essential oil
- 1 drop coriander essential oil

- 1/4 cup olive oil

Prepare dehydrator at 115 degrees F, or preheat oven to 200 degrees F. Wash kale and pat dry with paper towels; place in large bowl. Combine remaining ingredients in blender bowl and blend smooth 2 minutes. Pour on and massage in kale. Dehydrate until crisp or bake over an hour until crisp.

## GRILLED HALIBUT OR SALMON

Essential oils add such great flavor!

- 4 halibut or salmon fillets
- 1 Tablespoon olive oil
- 10-12 drops lime essential oil
- 6 drops black pepper essential oil
- 2 drops cilantro essential oil
- 3 cloves garlic, pressed
- Salt

In small bowl, combine olive oil, essential oils and garlic. Pat on fillets to coat, then sprinkle with salt. Preheat grill to medium heat and grill until just tender.

## HEARTY LENTIL STEW

You will be surprised at how tasty this is!

- 6 cups water
- 1 cup dry lentils
- 1 medium-small onion, diced
- 3 cloves garlic, minced
- 3 med/large potatoes, washed and diced
- 2 Tablespoons Braggs liquid aminos
- 1 1/2 teaspoon salt
- 1 drop oregano essential oil
- 1/4 cup chopped cilantro
- 4 large handfuls spinach leaves (baby or torn)

In large pot, combine water, lentils, onions, and garlic; simmer 45 minutes. Add potatoes and seasonings and simmer another 15 minutes, adding more water if necessary. Remove from heat and stir in remaining ingredients. Serve with carrot and celery sticks.

## CRUSTLESS QUICHE

No crust to mess with, great main dish with a green salad side!

- 3 large Anaheim chili, diced
- 1/2 red onion, diced
- 1 Tablespoon coconut oil
- 1 cup torn spinach or kale
- 1 1/2 cups coconut milk
- 1/3 cup raw cashews
- 5 eggs
- 3/4 teaspoon salt
- 1 drop coriander or cilantro essential oil
- 1 drop rosemary essential oil

Preheat oven to 375 degrees F. Dice chili and onion and place in pie plate with coconut oil in oven to soften and sizzle while preparing other ingredients. Prepare spinach or kale; set aside. In blender combine remaining ingredients and blend 2 minutes. Remove pie plate, spread on spinach or kale, and pour on egg mixture. Bake 20-25 minutes.

## CHICKEN FAJITAS

One of our favorite meals!

- 2 large chicken breasts, cut into strips
- 1/8 teaspoon salt
- 1 drop black pepper or coriander essential oil
- 3 drops lime or lemon essential oil
- 3 cloves garlic, minced
- 1 Tablespoon olive oil
- 1 medium yellow or red onion, sliced in 1/4 inch strips
- 1 large red pepper, cut into 1/4 inch strips
- 2 green chili peppers, cut into 1/4 inch strips
- Non-GMO corn tortillas

- Spicy Guacamole
- Fresh Mexican Salsa
- Shredded green leaf lettuce

In large bowl, combine chicken with oils and salt. Marinate 2-3 hours if time allows. Heat wok or skillet, salute chicken in coconut oil until mostly cooked through. Add onion, red pepper and green chili and sauté on medium. Meanwhile warm tortillas lightly and prepare other ingredients. Line open tortilla with chicken mixture; top with condiments, then roll up tortillas. For variation: use Romaine lettuce for the wraps instead of the tortillas.

## BLACK BEAN RICE STACKS

A simple meal, colorful, filling, and satisfying!

- 1 1/2 cup brown rice
- 6 cups cooked black beans (with liquid)
- 1 Tablespoon hot red pepper sauce
- 2 drops coriander essential oil
- 1 teaspoon salt (less if beans are salted)
- 2 avocados, diced
- 2 red bell peppers, diced
- 2 ears non-GMO corn, cut off cob
- 6 green onions, chopped
- Chopped red or green leaf lettuce
- 1/2 cup fresh chopped cilantro

In medium saucepan, bring 4 1/2 cups water to boiling and add rice. Turn heat down to simmering, don't stir, simmer 30-35 minutes, turn off heat, and place on the lid until ready. Meanwhile, combine beans, hot pepper sauce, oil and salt in saucepan and heat. Prepare raw vegetables as suggested. To serve, mound the rice on individual plates, spoon on black bean mixture, and top with generous portions of vegetables as desired. Top with red pepper sauce if desired!

## GRANOLA-YOGURT PARFAITS

Yummy for breakfast or dessert!

- 1 pint unsweetened vanilla coconut milk yogurt
- 3 drops wild orange essential oil
- 2 cup crunchy granola, made with clean ingredients
- 1/2 cup slivered or sliced almonds, or chopped pecans
- 2-3 cups fresh prepared fruit (raspberries, blueberries, diced bananas)

Add essential oil to yogurt. In parfait glasses or small cups, layer fruit, granola, then yogurt, top with nuts. Repeat and Enjoy!

## ORANGE-VANILLA ICE DELICIOUS

A family favorite for sure!

- 2 cans coconut milk (regular, not lite)
- 3/4 cup honey
- or 1/2 cup honey
- and 1/2 teaspoon clear liquid stevia
- 1/8 teaspoon salt
- 1 teaspoon xanthan gum
- 2 teaspoons vanilla
- 8 drops wild orange essential oil
- 1 can more pure cold water

In blender bowl place 2 cans coconut milk. Add all remaining ingredients except last water. Blend at least 1 minute, then stir in water. Chill first, if desired, then proceed according to ice cream maker's directions. Recipe makes approximately 2 quarts of Ice Delicious.

This is a basic recipe for Ice Delicious. For variation, decrease water and add 2-3 cups berries or other fruits. Lemon essential oil can also be substituted.

# Chapter 31

# CLEANSING PRODUCTS WITH ESSENTIAL OILS

## You Can Make Most Any Cleaning Product with These Few Simple Ingredients

- Baking soda
- Borax
- Liquid Castile soap
- Cream of tartar
- Diatomaceous earth
- Essential oils
- Washing soda
- White vinegar
- Soap flakes or Zote soap

## Most Common Essential Oils Suggestions

- Bergamot
- Grapefruit
- Lavender
- Lemon
- Lemongrass
- Lime
- Melaleuca
- Orange
- Rosemary
- Wintergreen

## GLASS AND MIRROR CLEANER

- 1/2 cup white vinegar
- 1/2 cup water
- 2 drops lemon essential oil

Put in 8 oz. glass spritzer bottle, wipe with paper towels.

## GUM OR GUM RESIN REMOVER

- lemon essential oil
- warm water and soap

Apply essential oil, and then follow with hot soap and water rinse.

## BATHROOM DISINFECTANT

- 2 drops each: clove, cinnamon, orange, eucalyptus, rosemary (or melaleuca)
- 8 oz. water in 8 oz. spritzer bottle

Cleaning product will:

- disinfect counter tops
- clean tile
- disinfect and wipe down toilet
- disinfect floors (several squirts with a wet water mop
- freshen air
- sanitize hands
- work as a mouth spritzer / rinse

## FRUIT AND VEGGIE WASH

- 2 drops each: clove, cinnamon, orange, eucalyptus, rosemary (or melaleuca)
- 8 oz. water in 8 oz. spritzer bottle

Spritz on produce then rinse thoroughly.

## CAR DISINFECTANT

Pour Fruit and Veggie Wash into a 2 oz. glass spritzer. Keep inside the car in the console and use as:

- Hand sanitizer
- Air freshener and disinfectant (especially when someone is coughing)
- Mouth spritzer

## LAUNDRY STAIN REMOVER

- 1 Tablespoon cream of tartar
- 2 drops lemon essential oil
- Few drops water

Combine to make a paste. Apply to the stain and allow the paste to set or dry completely before washing.

## DRYER SHEETS

- 5" square scraps of cotton cloth
- 2 drops lavender, wild orange, chamomile or other essential oil

Wet cloth with water; drop on oil and add to dryer with clothes. Reuse cloths time and time again.

## WALL CLEANER

- 1 cup water
- 1/2 cup white vinegar
- 6 lemon or grapefruit essential oil

Combine in a glass spray bottle; spray on walls and wipe down with cloth.

## DRAIN CLEANER

- 1 cup baking soda
- 1 cup white vinegar

- 3 drops melaleuca essential oil
- 1 large pot of boiling water

Place these in sink in order given. Works well.

## TILE CLEANER

- Baking soda
- White vinegar
- Clove and melaleuca essential oils

Sprinkle on soda; spray with vinegar, add essential oils to disinfect and fight mold. Scrub with a green scrubber – works great!

## TOILET BOWL CLEANER

- 1/2 cup baking soda or borax
- 1/2 cup white vinegar
- 2 drops eucalyptus or lemon essential oils

Pour in each toilet; scrub lightly with toilet brush.

## OVEN CLEANER

It's nice to know one can be non-toxic.

- 1 16-oz box baking soda
- 1/2 cup salt
- 1/4 cup borax or washing soda
- 1/4 cup water
- 10 drops lemon or lemongrass essential oil
- 5 drops rosemary essential oil
- White vinegar

Combine first 6 ingredients to make a paste; spread inside oven. Heat to 250° for 15 minutes. Spray on white vinegar; wipe down, rinse well.

## CREAMY SOFT SCRUBBER

- 1/2 cup baking soda

- Liquid Castile soap
- 1 teaspoon vegetable glycerin
- 1-2 drops each melaleuca and lemon essential oils

Combine in bowl in order given and mix to make a paste. Store it in a sealed glass jar.

## SINK CLEANSER

- Baking soda
- White vinegar

Sprinkle on soda, spray on white vinegar, wash with dish cloth.

# Chapter 32

# BODY CARE
# WITH ESSENTIAL OILS

## ULTIMATE SKIN PROTECTION OIL

- 2 oz. fractionated coconut oil (solid parts remove to remain liquid)
- 20 drops pure lavender essential oil
- 8 drops pure helichrysum essential oil
- 2 drops pure rose essential oil (optional)

Place in 2 oz. glass or amber oil container with drip cap or spritzer top. Apply before going out in the sun for periods longer than 15-20 minutes. Apply after being out in the sun, adding lavender essential oils for a burn.

## LIP BALM

- 2 Tablespoons olive oil
- Scant 1 teaspoon bees wax beads
- 20 drops lavender, ylang, orange/peppermint essential oils (pick your flavor)

Melt oil and bees was beads on stove in small saucepan just until wax melts. Drop in essential oils of choice. Divide in 3 containers or pour into tubes and allow it to set up before disturbing.

## MELALEUCA SALVE

Follow the Lip Balm recipe substituting 30 drops melaleuca oil for the other essential oils. Excellent for cold sores, chapped lips, wounds, or cuts.

## BATH SALTS

- 2 cups Epsom Salt or Sea Salt
- 15-20 drops essential oils:
- **Relaxing**: lavender or Roman chamomile essential oil
- **Energizing**: wild orange, grapefruit essential oils
- **Drawing/viruses**: peppermint, eucalyptus & melaleuca essential oils (10-12 drops each)
- **Fevers**: peppermint essential oil

Combine in a jar with a tight lid. Use 1/3 to 1/2 cup of salts per bath. If you want to absorb the oils, keep the water cooler; if you want to draw out toxins, keep the water as warm as possible. To pull down a fever, keep the water cooler than warm, but not cold.

## TOOTH POWDER

- 2 Tablespoons calcium supplement powder (can open capsules)
- 1 Tablespoon baking soda
- 1 teaspoon salt
- 1/4 teaspoon powdered stevia or 1 drop clear liquid (opt.)
- 6-8 drops of peppermint, wintergreen, clove, and/or cinnamon essential oil

Mix well; spoon into a container with a squirt tip for use. This tooth powder may be different than using a paste, but it is very good. Baking soda is a very good teeth cleanser.

# ABOUT THE AUTHOR

Over 30 years ago, while experiencing several health challenges, Erleen Tilton was introduced to a naturopathic physician who introduced her to a system. This system of whole foods, cleanses, quality nutritional supplements, and nature's medicines brought her renewed, energetic health within a short few months. From there she began her journey as a passionate wellness educator and has achieved titles as Holistic Nutritionist, Certified Aroma Therapist, Certified Holistic Wellness Coach, and Author of over 12 other wellness books and publications.

Erleen's greatest passion is to help people transform their lives as they learn the secrets of wellness that are found in nature! Her mission is to help others learn, then live the healthy, abundant life as well as joint venture with many others who are also passionate about nature's wellness, so together they can lift the lives of many people all over the globe to a greater degree of wellness!

Erleen's greatest love is her family. She partners and travels with her husband, Bill, in their wellness pursuits; she has six children, and currently thirteen grandchildren. She loves family time, quilting, gardening, plant identification, and hiking at their mountain home.

# REFERENCES

[1] *Modern Essentials*, Aroma Tools, 6th edition, pg. 3

[2] https://myoilbusiness.wordpress.com/2014/04/15/essential-oils-and-the-bible/myoilbusiness.wordpress.com, pg. 3

[3] *Traditional Foods are Your Best Medicine,* Ronald F. Schmid, N.D., pg. 17

[4] National Mental Health Association, pg. 18

[5] *The Garden of Eating: A Produce-dominate Diet & Cookbook,* Rachel Albert-Matesz, pg. 20

[6] http://www.aacap.org/App_Themes/AACAP/docs/facts_for_families/79_obesity_in_children_and_teens.pdf, www.aacap.org, March 2011, pg. 24

[7] http://teens.webmd.com/teens-plastic-surgery, www.teens.webmd.com, pg 24

[8] *Perfect Weight America*, Jordan Rubin, pg. 26

[9] *Perfect Weight America*, Jordan Rubin, pg. 27

[10] www.mayoclinic.org, http://www.mayoclinic.org/healthy-living/nutrition-and-healthy-eating/in-depth/fiber/art-20043983, pg. 28

[11] http://www.cancerfightingstrategies.com/ph-and-cancer.html#sthash.Iy1SAFZi.dpbs, www.cancerfightingstrategies.com, pg. 31

[12] http://www.trans4mind.com/nutrition/pH.html, www.trans4mind.com, pg. 31

[13] ibid, pg. 32

[14] https://www.aspca.org/fight-cruelty/farm-animal-cruelty/cows-factory-farms, pg. 34

[15] www.news-medical.net, pg. 34

[16] http://modernsurvivalblog.com/health/high-orac-value-antioxidant-foods-top-100/, pg. 39

[17] www.bragg.com, http://bragg.com/blog/index.php/all-natural-organic-whole-live-foods/bragg-organic-apple-cider-vinegar-featured-in-livestrong-article, pg. 40

[18] http://www.healthline.com/health/diabetes/insulin-and-glucagon#Overview1, www.healthline.com, pg. 43

[19] http://breakingmuscle.com/nutrition/insulin-and-glucagon-how-to-manipulate-them-and-lose-fat, pg. 43

[20] ibid, pg. 44

[21] http://www.rense.com/general86/ppos.htm, pg. 53

[22] "The Improvement Era", March 1948, pg. 53

[23] Ibid, pg. 53

[24] http://www.dailymail.co.uk/health/article-2861523/How-children-eating-70-teaspoons-sugar-day-Try-make-family-follow-healthy-diet-experiment-shock-you.html, pg. 53

[25] *Perfect Weight America,* Jordan Ruben, pg. 54

[26] http://www.rense.com/general86/ppos.htm, pg. 55

[27] http://www.seattleorganicrestaurants.com/vegan-whole-food/Pepsi-Coca-Cola-harmful-ingredients.php, pg. 56

[28] "The Energy Drink Epidemic", Thomas J. Boud, MD, Ensign Magazine, December 2008, pg. 56

[29] http://www.niaaa.nih.gov/alcohol-health/alcohols-effects-body, pg. 56

[30] Practice Prevention article, no reference, see studies of Herbert Needleman M.D., pg. 57

[31] http://groovygreenlivin.com/unacceptable-levels-a-film-about-the-chemicals-in-our-bodies-and-how-they-got-there/, pg. 58

[32] http://isthmusacupuncture.com/wp-content/uploads/2012/10/Cosmetic-and-Your-Health-Why-This-Matters.pdf, www.ewg.org, pg. 58

[33] http://www.aarp.org/health/drugs-supplements/info-08-2010/toxic-drugs-when-medicine-makes-you-sick.html, pg. 59

[34] www.livestrong.org http://www.livestrong.com/article/182003-what-are-the-dangers-of-plastic-bags-for-food-storage, pg. 60

[35] "Microwaving Your Food Isn't Safe", Larry Cook, pg. 61

[36] http://www.chemtrailcentral.com/ubb/Forum3/HTML/000226.html, pg. 62

[37] *Water: for Health, for Healing, for Life,* Batmanghelidj, MD (New York:

Warner Books, 2003) 225-226, pg. 71

[38] *Your Body's Many Cried for Water* by F. Batmanghelidj, MD, Second Edition, pgs. 13, 33, 41, 51, 56-57, 122, pg. 71

[39] http://articles.mercola.com/sites/articles/archive/2014/05/05/oil-pulling-coconut-oil.aspx, pg. 85

[40] *Food and Behavior*, Barbara Reed Stitt, pg. 91

[41] ibid, pg. 91

[42] ibid, pg 92

[43] http://www.feingold.org/PF/wisconsin1.html and http://raw-pleasure.com.au/latest/study-healthier-food-radically-improves-kids-lives, pg. 93

[44] ***Discover Magazine***, November 2006, "DNA is Not a Destiny", by Ethan Watters, pg. 95

[45] Worthington et al. (From UK Soil Association Fact Sheet). Journal of Complimentary Medicine 7:2161- 2163 (2001), pg. 95

[46] Dr. David Stewart, Ph.D., http://healthimpactnews.com/2013/why-essential-oils-heal-and-drugs-dont, pg. 109

[47] ibid, pg. 109

[48] Ibid, pg. 110

[49] *Modern Essentials*, Aroma Tools, pgs. 11-14, pg. 111

[50] Bob Wilson, www.autoenglish.org, Plants are People, http://www.autoenglish.org/listening/peoplereplants.htm, pg. 117

[51] Natural News, http://www.naturalnews.com/022652_vaccine_child_vaccines.html#ixzz3UKvClkZC, pg. 123

[52] *Vaccines: Are They Really Safe and Effective?*, Neil Z. Miller, updated February 1994, page 13, pg. 124

[53] Shirley's Wellness Cafe, http://www.shirleys-wellness-cafe.com/vaccines.htm, dr. Boyd Haley, Professor and Chair, Dept. of Chemistry, University of Kentucky, 2001, pg. 124

[54] www.organicconsumers.org, https://www.organicconsumers.org/news/how-toxic-are-your-household-cleaning-supplies, pg. 146

[55] www.aromatheraynaturals.com, http://www.aromatherapynaturals.com/pages/dangers-of-chemical-cleaners, pg 146

[56] ibid, pg. 147

[57] www.organicconsumers.org,
https://www.organicconsumers.org/news/how-toxic-are-your-household-cleaning-supplies, pg. 147

[58] Ibid, pg. 147

[59] http://www.rodalenews.com/unacceptable-levels-documentary, pg. 149

[60] www.panna.org, http://www.panna.org/issues/food-agriculture/pesticides-on-food, pg. 150

[61] http://www.foodsafetynews.com/2014/09/environmental-health-groups-want-epa-decision-on-toxic-pesticide-chlorpyrifos/, pg. 150

[62] *The Encyclopedia of Healing Foods*, Michael Murray N.D., Joseph Pizzorno, N.D., Laura Pizzorno, M.A., L.M.T., Atria Books, New York, pg. 151

[63] *Unacceptable Levels of Chemicals,* Leah Zerbe, pg. 154

[64] Ibid, pg. 154

[65] http://www.livestrong, http://www.livestrong.com/article/183108-toxins-in-skin-care/, pg. 155

[66] ibid, pg. 156

[67] http://www.ewg.org/2014sunscreen/the-trouble-with-sunscreen-chemicals/, pg. 156

[68] www.biospiritual-energy-healing.com and http://www.biospiritual-energy-healing.com/essential-oils-affect-our-minds.html, pg. 169

[69] *Emotions and Essential Oils*, Enlighten Alternative Healing, LLC, PO Box 1444, American Fork, UT 84003, pg. 171

[70] "Your Wish is Your Command" CD series, Kevin Trudeau, pg. 172

[71] The Holy Bible, King James version, pg. 173

[72] "Your Wish is Your Command" CD series, Kevin Trudeau, pg. 173

[73] www.drsirus.com, http://drsircus.com/medicine/function-vagus-nerve, pg. 181

[74] www.scientificamerican.com or http://www.scientificamerican.com/article/gut-second-brain, pg. 181

[75] www.drsirus.com, http://drsircus.com/medicine/function-vagus-nerve, pg. 182